Katharina Christina Wirnitzer

bikeeXtreme

Katharina Christina Wirnitzer

bikeeXtreme

Performance determining factors and vegan nutrition pattern to successfully complete the Transalp Challenge

Südwestdeutscher Verlag für Hochschulschriften

Impressum/Imprint (nur für Deutschland/ only for Germany)
Bibliografische Information der Deutschen Nationalbibliothek: Die Deutsche Nationalbibliothek verzeichnet diese Publikation in der Deutschen Nationalbibliografie; detaillierte bibliografische Daten sind im Internet über http://dnb.d-nb.de abrufbar.
Alle in diesem Buch genannten Marken und Produktnamen unterliegen warenzeichen-, marken- oder patentrechtlichem Schutz bzw. sind Warenzeichen oder eingetragene Warenzeichen der jeweiligen Inhaber. Die Wiedergabe von Marken, Produktnamen, Gebrauchsnamen, Handelsnamen, Warenbezeichnungen u.s.w. in diesem Werk berechtigt auch ohne besondere Kennzeichnung nicht zu der Annahme, dass solche Namen im Sinne der Warenzeichen- und Markenschutzgesetzgebung als frei zu betrachten wären und daher von jedermann benutzt werden dürften.

Verlag: Südwestdeutscher Verlag für Hochschulschriften Aktiengesellschaft & Co. KG
Dudweiler Landstr. 99, 66123 Saarbrücken, Deutschland
Telefon +49 681 37 20 271-1, Telefax +49 681 37 20 271-0, Email: info@svh-verlag.de
Zugl.: Innsbruck, Leopold-Franzens-Universität, Diss., 2009

Herstellung in Deutschland:
Schaltungsdienst Lange o.H.G., Berlin
Books on Demand GmbH, Norderstedt
Reha GmbH, Saarbrücken
Amazon Distribution GmbH, Leipzig
ISBN: 978-3-8381-0912-1

Imprint (only for USA, GB)
Bibliographic information published by the Deutsche Nationalbibliothek: The Deutsche Nationalbibliothek lists this publication in the Deutsche Nationalbibliografie; detailed bibliographic data are available in the Internet at http://dnb.d-nb.de.
Any brand names and product names mentioned in this book are subject to trademark, brand or patent protection and are trademarks or registered trademarks of their respective holders. The use of brand names, product names, common names, trade names, product descriptions etc. even without a particular marking in this works is in no way to be construed to mean that such names may be regarded as unrestricted in respect of trademark and brand protection legislation and could thus be used by anyone.

Publisher:
Südwestdeutscher Verlag für Hochschulschriften Aktiengesellschaft & Co. KG
Dudweiler Landstr. 99, 66123 Saarbrücken, Germany
Phone +49 681 37 20 271-1, Fax +49 681 37 20 271-0, Email: info@svh-verlag.de

Copyright © 2009 by the author and Südwestdeutscher Verlag für Hochschulschriften Aktiengesellschaft & Co. KG and licensors
All rights reserved. Saarbrücken 2009

Printed in the U.S.A.
Printed in the U.K. by (see last page)
ISBN: 978-3-8381-0912-1

In loving memory of Ada.

She always kept me modest
and never let me forget what really counts in life.

DEDICATION

Dedicated to the weakest and most helpless individuals on the earth,
the animals abused and brutally tortured
in the experimental laboratories of scientific and medical institutions,
as well as in the pharmaceutical and chemistry industries,
for whom only death brings salvation and release.

Foreword

by Franco M. Impellizzeri, Senior Research Fellow at the Neuromuscular Research Laboratory at Schulthess Klinik (Zürich, Switzerland), scientific advisor to the Interuniversity Research Center in Bioengineering and Sport Science of Rovereto (Italy) and scientific advisor to the Italian Cycling Federation Medical Commission, the most experienced researcher in the field of mountainbike sports and is the author of many leading publications focussed on this specific theme.

It is a great pleasure for me to introduce this book written by a talented "new" researcher who I hope will continue to contribute to increasing the body of knowledge about this and other fields of sport science. Mountainbiking is a popular recreational and competitive sport, as well as being an Olympic discipline since the Summer Olympic Games of Atlanta 1996. Despite its popularity, relatively few studies have investigated mountainbiking. Conducting a literature search on PubMed, before 2000, only about 20 publications examined aspects related to mountainbiking and, excluding the studies on injury–related topics, only a few addressed issues such as nutrition and physiology. In recent years, fortunately, mountainbiking has attracted the interest of sport scientists, and a still small but growing number of physiological studies have been published. Performing the same search on PubMed from 2001 to present about 40 papers can be retrieved, which reflects this increase in interest. However, less than 10 have examined the physiological aspects of mountainbiking. Therefore, it is clear that more research is needed.

The present book summarizes the findings of previous studies on mountainbiking. However, in this book the results of very recent investigations are also presented. These studies are very important because they cover aspects which have not yet been addressed, such as the physiological load imposed by what is probably the most important international stage race (Transalp Challenge), and the nutritional strategy adopted by a vegan athlete. This book is not centred on elite athletes, as has been the case in most publications, but this makes the manuscript even more important from a practical point of view, given that mountainbiking is practised by a large number of amateur riders who are almost ignored by the scientific literature. For these reasons this book can be considered state–of–the–art research on mountainbiking and represents a handbook essential for sport scientists, coaches and riders in planning and understanding mountainbike activity. Of course, this book is not intended to provide definite answers but ... "Science Will Never Explain Everything: That is Why it is So Useful!" (Robert Ehrlich, Skeptic, 2007).

Franco M. Impellizzeri, Bsc, MSc, PhD

Preface

This book represents a slightly modified and extended version of the successfully submitted thesis presented to the Faculty of Psychology and Sport Science (University of Innsbruck, Austria) in partial fulfillment of the requirements for the degree of doctor of science within the framework of the author`s thesis project. As such, it depicts an complete overview of the thesis project "bike*Xtreme*".

Mountainbiking, also called off–road cycling, is still a young and developing sports, compared to road cycling. Just as the Tour de France is the ultimate multiple day event for professional road cyclists, so the Transalp Challenge (TAC) is one of the most difficult mountainbike stage races in the world. The author aimed to investigate the TAC 2004 for the first time ever since the TAC was launched in 1998.

The author herself participated in and finished the TAC twice in 2003 and 2004. The successful completion of the TAC 2003, and the experience of the passion of extreme stage racing, led to both the initiation of "bike*Xtreme*" and the participation in the TAC 2004.

The "bike*Xtreme*" schedule consisted of the following:

- ✓ Preparation of the project (1st October 2003 – 31st March 2004): broad as well as deep review of the literature available relating to mountainbike sports.
- ✓ Start of project on 1st April 2004: Design and organisation of the field study as the core of data source.
- ✓ Completion of the field study (16th – 24th July 2004: subsequently described in detail in this book) performed under the authentic race burden of the TAC 2004, officially held during 17th – 24th July 2004.
- ✓ Collection of data sets recorded by subjects (25th July – 30th September 2004).
- ✓ Evaluation and analysis of data with only complete sets.
- ✓ Presentation and promotion of results and findings at international scientific meetings and congresses in the area of Sport Science over the period of 2005 – 2008.
- ✓ Publications in interntional peer–reviewed journals and publishers in the area of Sport Science, Sports Medicine and Physiology since 2005, continuing into 2009.
- ✓ Being awarded of Young Reseracher Award, category "Sport Training" (University of Prague, 2005), and of Doktoratsstipendium (University of Innsbruck, 2006).
- ✓ End of project was also the end of study on 21st April 2009.

Contents

Abstract 13

1. Introduction 15

   1.1. Motivation 15

   1.2. Historical overview 15

2. Method 19

   2.1. Subjects 21
      2.1.1. Questionnaire 22
      2.1.2. Exercise intensity 22
      2.1.3. Bioelectrical Impedance Analysis 22
      2.1.4. Haematological parameters 22
      2.1.5. Vegan nutrition pattern 23

   2.2. Incremental test 25

   2.3. Characteristics of the Transalp Challenge 2004 28

   2.4. Collection of field data 38
      2.4.1. Questionnaire 38
      2.4.2. Exercise intensity 39
      2.4.3. Bioelectrical Impedance Analysis 39
      2.4.4. Haematological parameters 41
      2.4.5. Vegan nutrition pattern 42

   2.5. Statistical analysis 44

3. Results 45

3.1. Questionnaire 45

3.2. Exercise intensity 48

3.3. Status of body water and haematology 53

3.4. Vegan nutrition pattern 55

4. Discussion 63

4.1. Physiological parameters 63
4.1.1. Physiological profile of the MTB athlete 63
4.1.2. Exercise Intensity 64
4.1.3. Body water pools and haematology 70
4.1.4. Prerequisites for the TAC 73

4.2. Bike handling mastery and race tactics 76

4.3. Nutritional strategies – Vegan nutrition pattern 78

4.4. Mood and mental capacity 95

5. Conclusion 96

References 97

Abstract

In general, knowledge is sparse in the area of mountainbike (MTB) sports because MTBing is still a young and developing sports, compared to road cycling. Therefore, only a few studies have been published.

Just as the Tour de France is the ultimate multiple day event for professional road cyclists, so the Transalp Challenge (TAC) is one of the most difficult MTB stage races in the world. Therefore, the purpose of the field study within the framework of the author's thesis project "bikee*Xtreme*" was to determine the course, distribution and changes of the following parameters, caused by the TAC 2004: Heart rate and Borg's rate of perceived exertion (both indicators of exercise intensity), body water compartments, selected blood parameters and nutrient intake (energy and fluid intake) including vegan nutrition pattern.

Only athletes who successfully finished the TAC 2004 and who recorded complete data sets comprised the basis of this study. All subjects were well endurance trained amateur athletes and were experienced at competing in MTB marathon races.

This investigation was the first to
i) study an extreme MTB stage race,
ii) determine the exercise intensity during one of the most important MTB stage races in the world, showing the TAC 2004 to be physiologically very demanding and heavily involving both the aerobic and anaerobic energy system,
iii) detect acute effects (decline in body water pools simultaneously with hemoconcentration), which probably occurred due to a combination of heat induced and exercise induced dehydration during the first stage of TAC 2004,
iv) describe long term adaptations (expansion in body water pools simultaneously with hemodilution), formerly shown to occur as a consequence of repeated strenuous endurance strains during the TAC 2004,
v) study a female athlete during this difficult multi–day MTB marathon race and
vi) report the dietary intake during the TAC 2004, showing that a well planned vegan diet can adequately meet the nutritional demands of severe MTB stage racing.

To the best of the author's knowledge there have no studies investigating MTB marathon races, 1–day cross–country marathon races or MTB stage races have yet been published. Moreover, well controlled long term studies assessing the effects of a vegan diet on an athlete's performance, in particular endurance performance, have not yet been conducted. Therefore, the results currently presented might be useful to design specific training programs and to develop appropriate nutritional strategies to sustain the physical demands of severe MTB marathon and MTB stage races.

1. Introduction

1.1. Motivation

In the late 1980s, at the age of 14, I was given my first mountainbike (MTB). From then on I was addicted to this new kind of cycling sport. At that time, to the best of my knowledge, I was one of about five female MTBers in my federal state. In the past decade I have participated in several regional, national and international MTB marathon races (lasting one or even several days). Due to my passion, my whole family adopted this sport as their favourite leisure time activity.

Based on my passion for MTB sports and a deep and broad review of MTB specific literature available – which is sparseat present – I decided to write my thesis about the most challenging multi–day MTB marathon race in the world, the Transalp Challenge (TAC), in the year 2004.

At the same time as undertaking my investigation in sports science, I reached the peak of my career as an MTB athlete by finishing the TAC 2004 with the final rank of 16th – I had never dreamt of exceeding my target of reaching the top 20.

1.2. Historical overview

In September 1976 a new kind of bicycle, the off–road bike or MTB, was created by four young men (Gary Fisher, Charly Kelly, Joe Breeze and Tom Ritchey) in California, USA (Gerig and Frischknecht 1996). The first MTB competitions were held in the early 1980s (Auferbauer 2007). Since then this new kind of cycling sports has grown rapidly. The first MTB World Championships to be officially recognized by the Union Cycliste Internationale (UCI) date back to 1990, with the first World Cup (WC) events having been held in 1991 (www.uci.ch).

The first MTB marathon ever held on 11th of August 1990 in Eschlikon (Switzerland), indicates the history of the long distance category. That event laid the foundation for the biggest mass movement in the history of MTBing and from then on the number of long distance events exploded, along with the number of starters in these MTB marathon events. In the mid 1990s riders were glad to grab a starting place (Lesewitz 2005). After Stefan Götz, Specialized (Lesewitz 2004): *"Marathon was probably the best idea for MTB sports. It covers the whole spread of this sport."*

Nowadays, MTB marathon is a public sport and a booming industry. There are about 120 MTB marathon events of all kinds listed in the race calendar, each with up to 10,000 participants (Lesewitz 2004). According to the UCI Rules (www.uci.ch/Modules/BUILTIN/getObject.asp?MenuId=MTkzNg&ObjTypeCode=FILE&type=FILE&id=34424&), MTB races are divided into three types of events (UCI Rules, Chapter I §1, p. 1): Cross–country (XC), downhill and stage races. XC marathons (XCM) generally cover a closed circuit of at least 60 km in distance and last at least 3 hours. The XCM discipline is a mass start event. There are narrow tracks, paths through forests, rocky paths and the riders even have to ford streams (www.uci.ch).

Usually one day MTB marathon races can be characterized according to the total load of the race: a classic MTB marathon covers about 2400 m in altitude difference along with a distance of about 60 km, whereas extreme and ultraendurance (> 4 hours: Peters 2003) MTB marathons cover altitude differences of 3500 m to 7000 m along with distances of 70 km to 200 km while light courses (for beginners) have about 1000 m in altitude difference and distances of about 25 km.

The UCI Race Calendar (UCI Rules, Chapter I §3, p. 3) includes the XCM World Championship (officially held first in 2003 in Switzerland), XCM European Championship (officially held first in 2002 in Austria), XCM WC series (UCI Rules, Chapter VIII, §1, p. 24–25, www.uci.ch/templates/UCI/UCI5/layout.asp?MenuId=MTUzNDI) and numerous other global series, XCM stage races and XCM one day races. XCM has not yet gained acceptance as an Olympic event yet.

In the summer of 1990, the two German MTBers Andi Heckmaier and Uli Stanciu (founder of the TAC) were the first to cross the Central Alps, independently of each other (Lesewitz 2004, Scheele 2008).

In July 1998, the first TAC took place, following the model of the Tour de France. It was conceived as a multi–day competitive event for double teams (due to safety considerations) of both professional and recreational MTBers across the Central Alps (Figure 1). The UCI General Rules for stage races are met (UCI Rules, Chapter II §1, p. 6–7, Chapter VI §1, p. 22–23, Chapter VIII §2, p. 24–27). Today, three decades after the birth of the off–road bike, the term "Alpentransversale" is the term which is googled most often by European MTBers (Auferbauer 2007) and annually thousands of riders cross the (Eastern and Western) Alps on several different routes (Lesewitz 2005).

The purpose of this field study within the authors's thesis project "bikee*Xtreme*" was to investigate the TAC for the first time in order to determine the athletic performance capacity of MTBers. Moreover, the identification of physiological parameters and factors which might determine or rather limit MTB performance whilst competing in the TAC 2004 was a specific objective of the study of this severe XCM stage race.

Figure 1. Course of Transalp Challenge 2004 (with permission from 27th July 2009) covering an altitude difference of 22500 m over a distance of 662 km, starting at Mittenwald/BRD (17th July 2004), passing through Tyrol/AUT and finishing at Riva del Garda/ITA (24th July 2004).

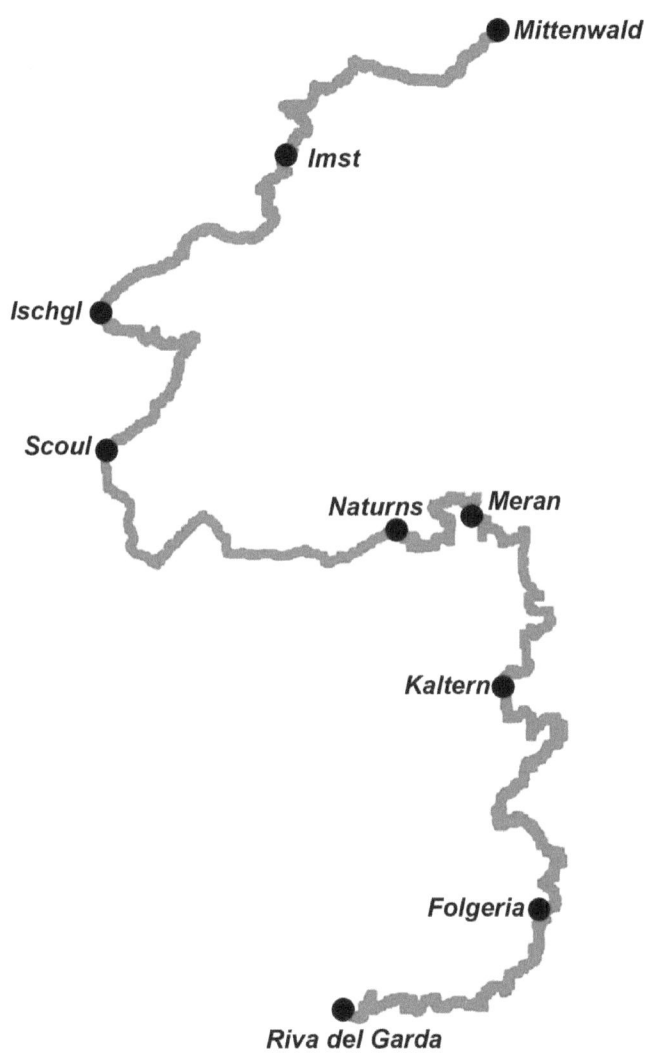

©Uli Stanciu www.bike–gps.com info@bike–gps.com

2. Method

The concept of conducting a field study under the authentic race burden of the TAC 2004 (Table 1) was supported by two researchers from the Australian Institute of Sport, Department of Physiology, who were working with Cadel Evans, formerly one of the worlds best MTBers and, to date, professional road cyclist at the Pro–Tour Team Silence–Lotto.

The design of this study was partly based on the work of, and a specific citation within, the Master Thesis "Competitive mountain bike and road cycling", Chapter 3, p. 69) of Hamilton Lee, Sport Physiologist (Lee 2003, with permission from 23rd May 2006):

"Laboratory studies conducted under constant exercise conditions hardly mimic the conditions encountered by competitive MTB cyclists in the field".

David T. Martin, Senior Sport Physiologist, whom I talked to after his invited speech "Cycling Power Output" at the Endurance Sport Science Conference, Birmingham, UK, 29 – 30 April 2006 (with permission from 18th July 2006), further advocated this choice of design:

"Laboratory testing of athletes can be a useful tool for assessing a number of physiological traits in a controlled condition. In some cases, the laboratory may be useful for establishing maximal performance abilities in a controlled environment that minimizes the influence of technique. However, when physiologists are working with athletes for a long time period in an attempt to improve their fitness for a special event it becomes important to work in the field. It is in the field where sports are really performed, under authentic conditions of training and competition (training–camps, worldcup–races, world championship and so on)."

Table 1. Methodical process of this study prior to and during the Transalp Challenge 2004. Baseline measurements were conducted for exercise intensity (laboratory testing), status of body water (BIA = Bioelectrical Impedance Analysis) and haematological parameters.

	Baseline	Stage 1	Stage 2	Stage 3	Stage 4	Stage 5	Stage 6	Stage 7	Stage 8
Questionnaire		x	x	x	x	x	x	x	x
Exercise intensity	x	x	x	x	x	x	x	x	x
BIA	x	x			x		x		
Haematological parameters	x	x			x		x		
Vegan nutrition survey		x	x	x	x	x	x	x	x

2.1. Subjects

The recruitment of participants for the study during the TAC 2004 occurred through the Internet forum of the TAC organizer and was carried out on a voluntary basis. 37 MTB athletes (from 10 nations) competing in the TAC 2004, were recruited for the study. Shortly before the start of this stage race, these athletes received information about the mode and schedule of the study, in order to become familiar with the process of measurement and to simplify the field study itself during the TAC 2004. Written informed consent was obtained after verbal and written explanation of the procedures. The investigation was approved by the Institutional Review Board (Department of Sport Science, University of Innsbruck, Austria) and performed according to the Declaration of Helsinki.

Given the technical and physical difficulties of a TAC, a large number of riders were enrolled in order to achieve a sufficient number of MTBers who would meet the inclusion criteria. Reasons for exclusion from the final analysis were mainly missed data due to breakdown or loss of heart rate (HR) monitors, sudden illness, aches and pains following an accident or tumble, drop out of competition or stolen bike. Only subjects who finished the TAC 2004 with complete data sets reported were included in the final analysis (Table 2). All of these remaining athletes were amateur cyclists and could be characterized as well endurance trained (classification adopted after Jeukendrup et. al. 2000) who were very experienced (four subjects had previously participated in the TAC, ranging from one to six successful finishes) MTBers. It can be presumed that, in the face of the extraordinary exertion caused by the overall load, the athletes who completed the TAC 2004 were in excellent physical shape.

When exclusively professional cyclists are studied the risk of obtaining falsified data influenced by any kind of doping should be considered. Direct comparison between professional and amateur MTB athletes would be preferable and is practicable as they usually participate in the same competitions. In general, however, professionals are not very keen to participate in such studies for several reasons, as was the case in this study (both professional MTBers, one a former multiple winner of the TAC, dropped out after the first stage of TAC 2004).

2.1.1. Questionnaire

The number of subjects involved in this set, who correctly filled out the daily questionnaire (Figure 2) varied on a daily basis due to several reasons. Further details are listed in Table 5.

2.1.2. Exercise intensity

7 subjects, 5 males (age: 34.7 ± 3.1 years, height: 1.71 ± 0.4 m, body mass: 63.3 ± 10.1 kg) and 2 females (age: 32.0 ± 2.8 years, height: 1.63 ± 0.02 m, body mass: 51 ± 1.4 kg), were included to quantify the exercise intensity throughout the whole period of TAC 2004.

2.1.3. Bioelectrical Impedance Analysis

13 subjects, 11 males (age: 32.6 ± 8.8 years, height: 1.78 ± 0.1 m, body mass: 72.4 ± 10.2 kg) and 2 females (age: 32.0 ± 2.8 years, height: 1.64 ± 0.04 m, body mass: 55.0 ± 7.1 kg), were included to determine the effects of fluid shifts in body water compartments caused by this MTB stage race.

2.1.4. Haematological parameters

6 subjects, 5 males (age: 29.0 ± 5.6 years, height: 1.82 ± 0.1 m, body mass: 74.6 ± 12.4 kg) and 1 female (age: 30 years, height: 1.61 m, body mass: 49 ± 1 kg) reliably not being doped, were included to determine acute shifts and long term adaptations in hemoglobin (Hb), hematocrit (Hct) and calculated plasma volume (PV_{CALC}).

2.1.5. Vegan nutrition pattern

1 female subject (age: 30 years, height: 1.61 m, body mass: 49 ± 1 kg) was recruited for this case report. The subject is a well experienced endurance off–road cyclist. In 2004 she started the TAC for the second time, having also previously finished the TAC before in 2003. To prepare for this eight–day stage race, the rider trained for between 20 – 25 hours a week for almost a year (including several ultraendurance MTB marathon races). The MTB used was a front suspension bike (10.2 kg). The female rider has successfully followed a vegan lifestyle (dietary pattern is determined to be exclusively based on a plant based nutrition, rejecting all products directly or indirectly from animal sources or tested on animals) as a daily routine as well as during endurance training and competition for five years (and to date, still continuing in 2009).

Table 2. Number of subjects remaining after the Transalp Challenge 2004 to build the basis of any specific data set. HR = heart rate. BIA = Bioelectrical Impedance Analysis.

	Total	male	female
Questionnaire	30 – 11	26 – 9	4 – 2
Exercise intensity (HR)	7	5	2
BIA	13	11	2
Haematological parameters	6	5	1
Vegan nutrition survey	1	–	1

Figure 2. Standard form of daily questionnaire (example).

Etappe/Stage: _3 – Ischgl -> Scuol_
No. and Name: _239/1 – Mustermann Peter_
Körpermasse/Bodymass: _74_ **kg**

Stimmung – mood

sehr gut / very good	gut / good	o.k.	schlecht / bad
☐	☐	☒	☐

Beine – muscles of legs

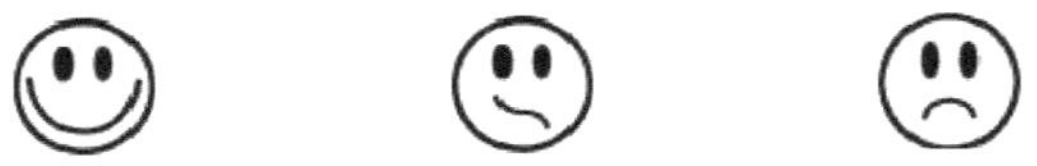

sehr gut / very good	o.k.		schlecht / bad
☐	☒		☐

BORG – RPE Skala
(Rate of perceived exertion)

6	keinerlei Anstrengung / not any exertion	☐
7		☐
7,5	sehr sehr leicht / extremely easy	☐
8		☐
9	sehr leicht / very easy	☐
10		☐
11	leicht / easy	☐
12		☐
13	etwas anstrengend / a little exertive	☐
14		☐
15	anstrengend / exertive	☐
16		☐
17	sehr anstrengend / very exertive	☐
18		☒
19	extrem anstrengend / extremely exertive	☐
20	maximal anstrengend / maximal exertive	☐

Wieviel Liter Flüssigkeit hast Du heute insgesamt getrunken?
How much litre of fluid have you drunken all over today? _4,5_ **lt.**

2.2. Incremental test

The subjects performed an incremental laboratory cycling test (set form: Figure 3) no more than seven days before the start of the TAC 2004. They were asked to avoid exhaustive exercise for at least 15 hours prior to testing. Tests were performed on an electromagnetically braked ergometer (Schoberer Rad Messtechnik SRM GmbH, Jülich, BRD). After 15 min of warm up with freely chosen workload and cadence, the test started at 100 W and workload was increased by 30 W every 5 min. The subjects were asked to maintain the cadence at 90 revolutions/minute (85 – 95 rpm: Takaishi et. al. 1996). The test was terminated upon voluntary exhaustion or incapacity to maintain a cadence around 90 rpm. When the last work load was not maintained for the full period peak power output (PPO) was calculated using the equation of Kuipers et. al. (1985): PPO = PO_{FINAL} + (t/300s x 30W), where PO_{FINAL} is the value for the last complete workload, 300 is the duration of the step in seconds, 30 W is the power output (PO) increment, and t is the time in seconds of the incomplete workload. In the last 30 s of each step, capillary blood samples (10 μL) were taken from the ear lobe and immediately analyzed (Vario Photometer, Diaglobal GmbH, Berlin, Germany). During the tests, HR and PO were continuously recorded.

Following similar previous studies on road cycling (stage races: Fernandez–Garcia et. al. 2000, Lucia et. al. 2003a+b, Lucia et. al. 1999, Padilla et. al. 2001, Palmer et. al. 1994, Rodriguez–Marroyo et. al. 2003; one day races: Neumayr et. al. 2002b/2003a/2004) and off–road cycling (Impellizzeri et. al. 2002/2005a, Lee et. al. 2002, Stapelfeldt et. al. 2004), the intensity zones were defined using the HR corresponding to the lactate thresholds (LTs). For each cyclist, the HR at a fixed concentration of 2 mmol/L (LT2) and 4 mmol/L (LT4) was determined. In addition, in order to obtain an exercise intensity zone which better reflects very high–demanding efforts, the HR at 6 mmol/L (LT6) was also measured. At and above this level energy supply is increasingly met by anaerobic sources (growing recruitment of type IIa fibres: Gilman and Wells 1993, Gilman 1996).

HR values at LTs were identified by straight line interpolation between the two closest points. From these data, four intensity zones were established to describe the profile of the TAC 2004:
1) LOW zone for intensity below the HR corresponding to LT2
2) MODERATE zone for intensity between the HR corresponding to LT2 and LT4
3) HIGH zone for intensity between the HR corresponding to LT4 and LT6
4) VERY HIGH zone for intensity above the HR corresponding to LT6.

Figure 3. Standard form of laboratory test protocol (example).

Laboratory test: Competitor TAC 04

Kind of performance-test: time and gradually step-increasment

Step duration (min)	Gradually step-increasment (Watt)	Your choice
every 5 min	increasing 30 Watt	X
every 3 min	increasing 20 Watt	

Threshold-data of your performance-test:

Lactat (mmol/L)	Heartrate HR (bpm)	Cycle-power-output per kg bodymass (Watt/kg)
2 mmol/L	148	3.01
4 mmol/L	163	3.56
6 mmol/L	170	3.83
Individual aerob-anaerobe threshold IAT	158	

Performance duration overall	35 min
Maximum Heartrate HR_{MAX} (bpm)	188
Maximum cycle-power-performance ($Watt_{MAX}$)	199
Maximum cycle-power-performance per kg bodymass ($Watt_{MAX}$/kg)	4.19

2.3. Characteristics of the Transalp Challenge 2004

1074 athletes (537 double teams, within the categories: Men, Masters, Mixed and Women, from nations all over the world) participated in the TAC 2004. The total altitude climbed was 22500 m and the total distance covered by the riders was 662 km. This resulted in a daily average altitude climbed of 2810 m and distance of 83 km. The longest uphill climb and downhill section as one unit was 1700 m and 1400 m in altitude difference, respectively. The total distance climbed uphill was 315 km and in downhill section it was 275 km. In terms of the daily total load, single stages can be compared to those of the mountainous Vuelta a Espana. Just as the Tour de France is the ultimate multiple day event for professional road cyclists, so the TAC is one of the most difficult XCM races in the world (Table 3). The drop out rate after eight consecutive stages of competition in 2004 was 18.81 %, also including professional riders.

The characteristics of the TAC 2004 are presented in Table 4. Peak values of temperature and relative humidity were taken from meteorological stations nearest to competitive waypoints of the TAC 2004 (ZAMG, Innsbruck, Austria). In particular, the course profile of Stages 1 to 8 is presented in Figures 4 – 11 in more detail (with permission from 24th October 2007).

Table 3. The three most important tours in road cycling and MTB sports.

Road Cycling	MTB
Giro d`Italia, ITA (May)	Cape Epic, SA (March)
Tour de France, FRA (July)	**Transalp Challenge, BRD/AUT/ITA (July)**
Vuelta a Espana, ESP (September)	Transrockies, USA (September)

Table 4. Characteristics and nature of course profile of the Transalp Challenge 2004.

	Unit	Stage 1	Stage 2	Stage 3	Stage 4	Stage 5	Stage 6	Stage 7	Stage 8	Mean (±SD)
Temperature	°C	28	24	24	29	32	33	28	22	28 (±4)
Humidity (relative)	%	45	45	44	50	45	60	50	94	69 (±17)
Stage distance	km	80	73	74	119	54	73	124	67	83 (±25)
Stage time (n=7)	min	307	349	286	415	279	289	443	289	326 (±61)
Stage time (n=1)	min	293	328	287	402	225	280	426	278	315 (±60)
Uphill cycling										
Total altitude climbed	m	2398	3099	2619	3366	2103	2732	3995	2141	2807 (±650)
Distance	km	43.8	43.9	39.7	46.3	23.1	34.7	69.1	14.7	39 (±16)
Downhill cycling										
Total altitude climbed	m	2512	2556	2770	4030	2333	2633	3264	3234	2917 (±560)
Distance	km	29.1	26.4	26.8	67.1	27.5	34.6	28.2	34.9	34 (±14)
Nature of course profile										
Asphalt	%	18.3	39.8	16.8	4.4	14.3	10.8	10.8	25	17.5 (±11)
Cycle track	%	8.1	20.2	24.5	32.6	26.6	40	60	25.3	29.7 (±15)
Gravel track/trail	%	51.1	27	54.3	52.1	32	29.2	19.3	34.1	37.4 (±13)
Forest–/meadow trail	%	18.3	5	1.2	3.3	16.9	8.8	7.6	0.5	7.7 (±7)
Alpine trail	%	4.2	8	1.6	7.4	10.2	9.7	2.3	15.1	7.3 (±5)
Push and/or carry	%	0	0	1.6	0.2	0	1.5	0	0	0.4 (±1)

Figure 4. Stage 1 (Mittenwald/BRD to Imst/AUT; with permission from 27th July 2009).

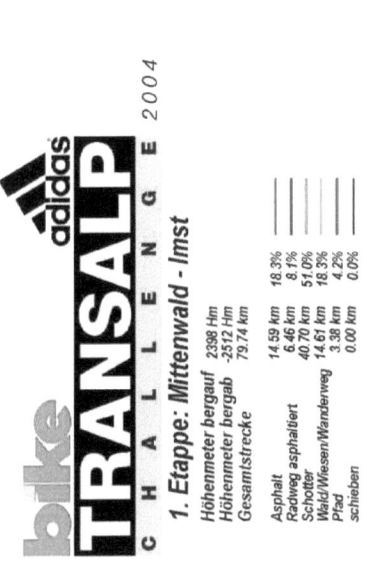
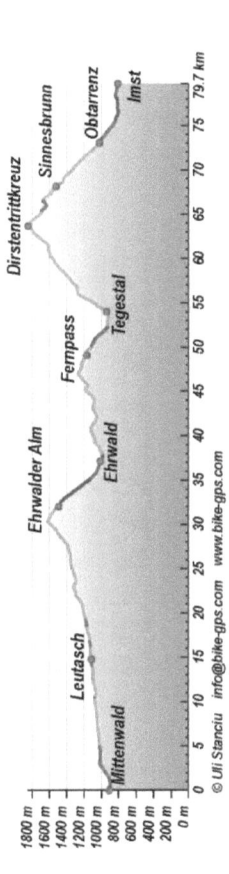

Figure 5. Stage 2 (Imst to Ischgl/AUT; with permission from 27th July 2009).

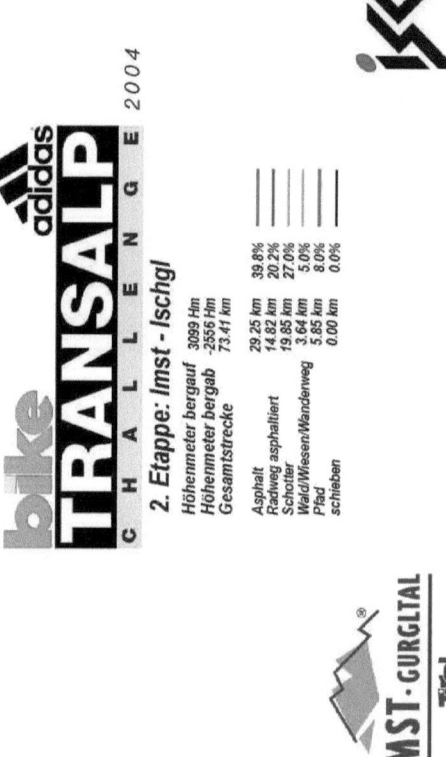
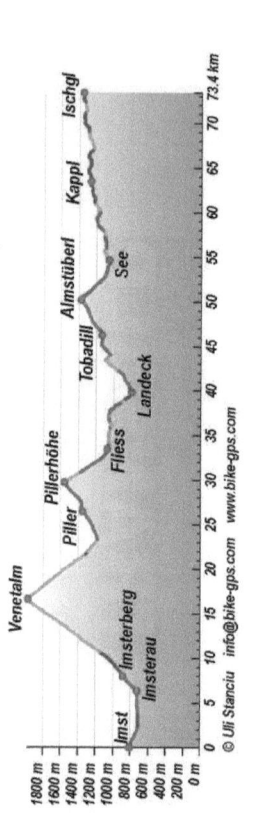

Figure 6. Stage 3 (Ischgl/AUT to Scuol/CH; with permission from 27th July 2009).

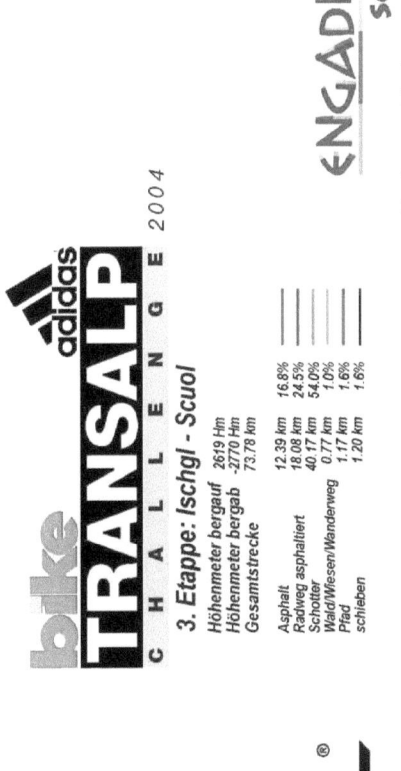

Figure 7. Stage 4 (Scuol/CH to Naturns/ITA; with permission from 27th July 2009).

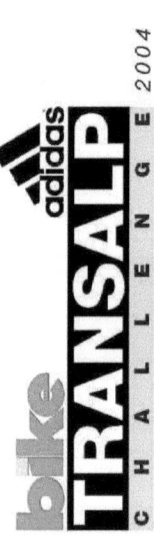
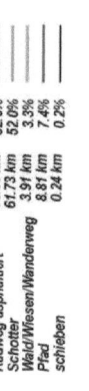
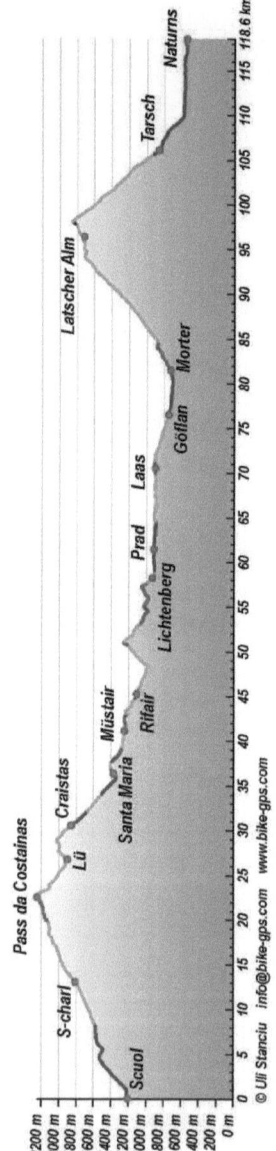

Figure 8. Stage 5 (Naturns to Meran/ITA; with permission from 27th July 2009).

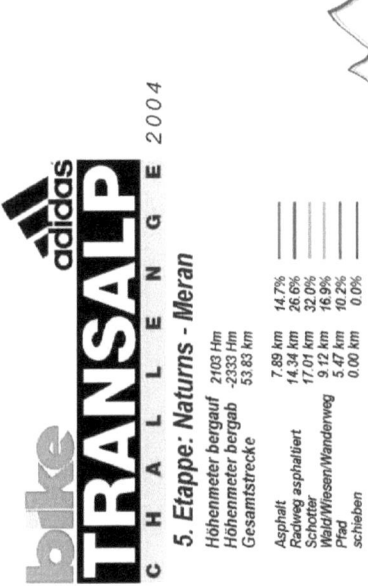
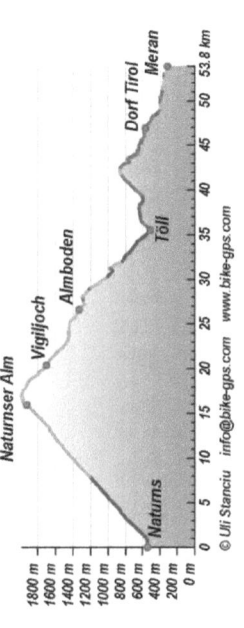

Figure 9. Stage 6 (Meran to Kaltern/ITA; with permission from 27th July 2009).

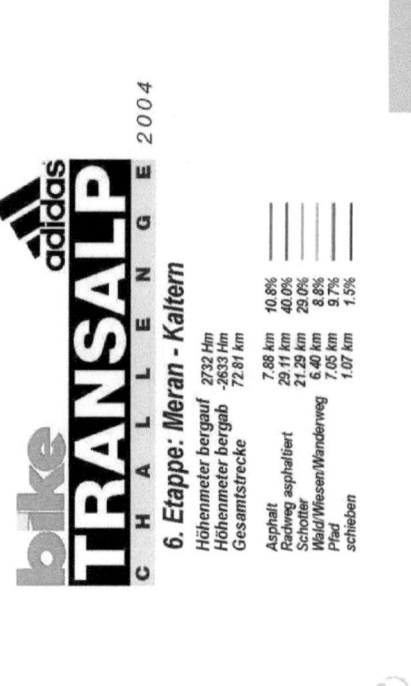
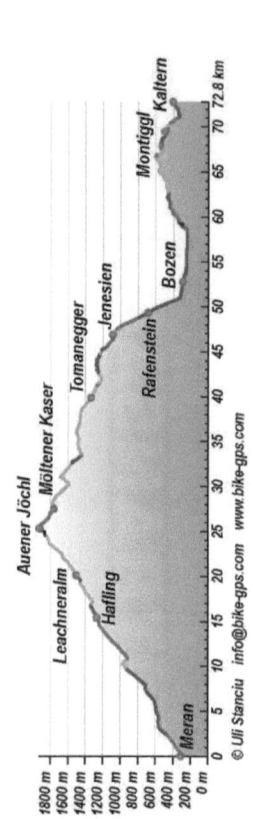

Figure 10. King size Stage 7 (Caldaro to Folgaria/ITA; with permission from 27th July 2009).

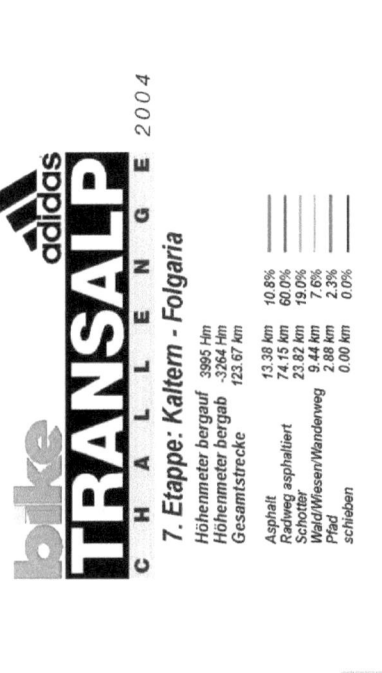
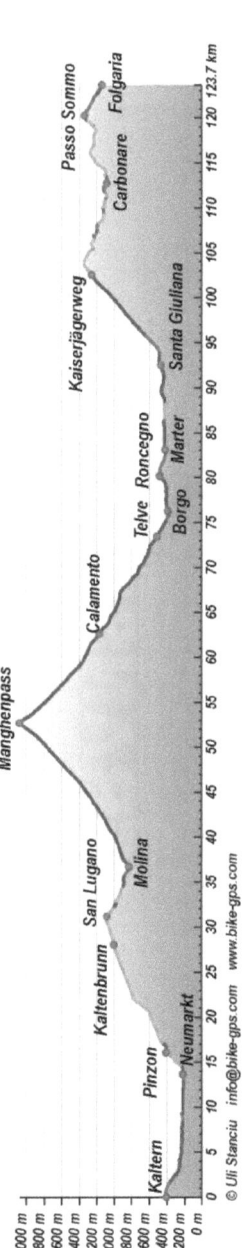

Figure 11. Stage 8 (Folgaria to Riva del Garda/ITA; with permission from 27th July 2009).

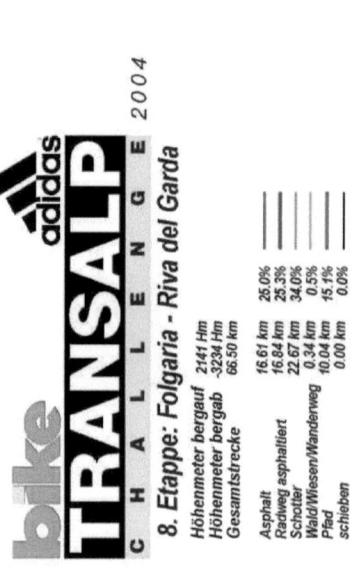
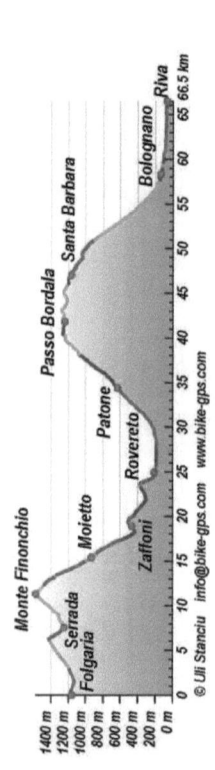

2.4. Collection of field data

The daily competition schedule varies to meet the organisational demands of 1074 MTBers (daily registration, early start time, late finish time, recovery stations, toilets, catering, accommodation, luggage and material transport, medical support, technical support and several more). In the light of the huge logistical and personal challenges of simply participating in the TAC 2004, it was difficult to conduct all the measurements of this field study. After the race, it was not possible to assemble the subjects on their first day of recovery to take a final body water and haematological measurement performed by equilibrated body water pools for understandable reasons, which included meeting their families after eight days of exhausting stage racing, sudden departures on homeward journeys and the immediate onset of vacations.

2.4.1. Questionnaire

Prior to the TAC 2004 athletes had been familiarized with the daily questionnaire. The 15 graded RPE (rate of perceived exertion) scale (Borg 1998) was used to facilitate the interpretation of HR data in order to quantify exercise intensity. The subjects were instructed to rate how hard each entire stage was by reporting the overall RPE after they had finished. Smilies were included to rate the status of athletes` mood and fatigue of leg muscles. This additional method of rating was chosen to motivate the subjects to reflect their level of mental and physical exertion. The cyclists were instructed to maintain adequate fluid and nutritional intake (high in carbohydrates). Fluid intake since breakfast and body mass were immediately reported after each individual finish of the daily stages. Body mass was measured including bike uniform but without MTB shoes (Medica, Soehnle, Germany).

2.4.2. Exercise intensity

HR has been frequently used to indirectly describe the exercise intensity during both road cycling (Fernandez–Garcia et. al. 2000, Lucia et. al. 1999/2000/2003a+b, Padilla et. al. 2001/2008, Palmer et. al. 1994, Rodriguez–Marroyo et. al. 2003) and MTB XC races (Impellizzeri et. al. 2002/2005a). In contrast to power profiles, HR of a specific type of exercise has been shown to have a more stable pattern (Hurst and Atkins 2002/2006, Stapelfeldt et. al. 2004), which is an advantage over the HR method.

Jeukendrup and Van Diemen (1998) suggested that HR might be a good marker of whole body stress while power output might be a better indicator of exercise intensity. On the other hand, according to Padilla et. al. (2008), since no indicators of exercise intensity free of potential limitations exist, the use of HR can be acceptable for quantifying the exercise intensity during cycling competitions. The author is absolutely aware that the use of HR method to determine the intensity of a specific event is potentially limited by various factors. However, duration of daily race, terrain, altitude (summits up to 3000 m), environmental conditions as well as the kind of bike (front suspension MTBs) are considered to be of limited importance in the HR response as they are constant for all subjects.

During the TAC 2004, the HR response was continuously monitored by using short range HR telemetry systems (S710, Polar Electro Oy, Kempele, Finland). The HR was recorded by using a sample rate of 60 s in order to be able to store the HR data of the entire MTB event. At the end of this stage race, all HR files were collected and downloaded. The recorded data was analysed with specific software (Polar Precision Performance 4 SW, Polar Electro Oy, Kempele, Finland) and HR files including more than 5 % of sample data outside a range of 60 – 220 beats/min (bpm) were excluded from the analysis. The relative intensity of exercise was expressed as a percentage of maximum HR reached in each stage ($HR_{MAX}Field$) and of laboratory determined maximum HR ($HR_{MAX}Lab$).

2.4.3. Bioelectrical Impedance Analysis (BIA)

After extensive validation, various authors have attested the BIA technique to be reliable in assessing body hydration status in healthy, euhydrated adults under standardized conditions (Buchholz et. al. 2004, Fellmann et. al. 1999, Grund et. al. 2001,

Koulmann et. al. 2000, Kyle et. al. 2004a+b, Mischler et. al. 2003, Nose et. al. 1988, O`Brien et. al. 2002, Pialoux et. al. 2004, Segal 1996, Thomas et. al. 1998) and for monitoring changes in body water pools within individuals over time (Buchholz et. al. 2004, Kyle et. al. 2004b, Shanholtzer and Patterson 2003).

The BIA 2000 M multifrequency bioelectrical impedancemeter (Data Input, Hofheim, Germany, NUTRI4 software package) was used to measure the distribution of compartmental body water. An arrangement of four electrodes was applied to the skin after alcohol preparation. The injector electrodes were placed (after users manual) just below the phalangeal–metacarpal joint in the middle of the dorsal side of the right hand and just below the transverse (metatarsal) arch on the superior/upper side of the right foot. Detector electrodes were placed on the posterior side of the right wrist, midline with the prominent pisiform bone on the medial (fifth phalangeal) side and ventrally across the medial ankle bone of the right ankle.

Baseline measurements of BIA were conducted in the morning before the start of the TAC 2004, at between 9 a. m. and 11 a. m. The subjects were asked to avoid exhaustive exercise for at least 15 hours prior to this baseline measurement. Post exercise data were respectively determined after 5 min of rest in a relaxed supine position, either immediately or within a maximum of 10 min after individual finish of Stages 1, 4 and 6.

Figure 12. BIA measurement post exercise, shown here after Stage 6 at Caldaro/ITA.

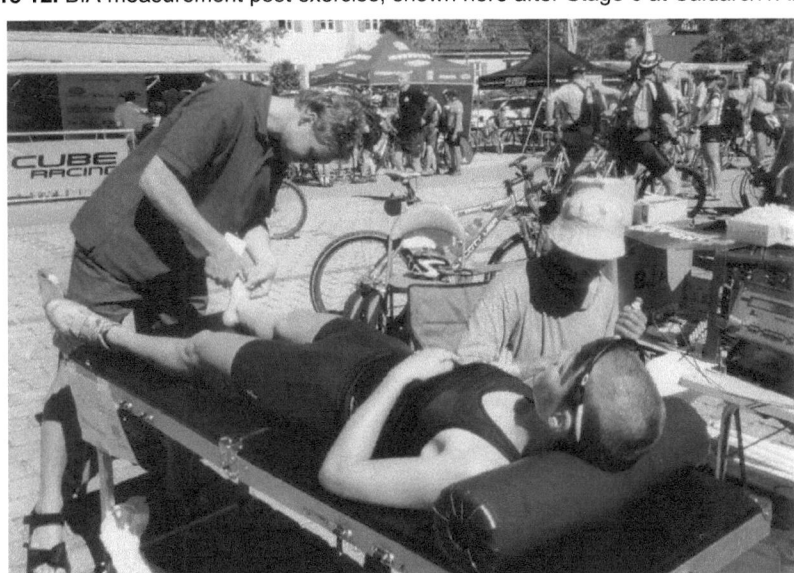

2.4.4. Haematological parameters

Blood samples (2 x 10 µL) based on capillary blood from the finger tip were drawn (measurement process as previously described in Chapter 2.4.3.) to detect Hb and Hct levels (Miniphotometer plus LP 20, Lange, Germany). Robinson et. al. (2005) ratified this method to reliably determine blood parameters in the field in absence of standardized laboratory conditions. Relative changes in PV_{CALC} ($\Delta\%PV$) were calculated from pre– and post exercise values of Hb and Hct according to the equation of Strauss et. al. (1951):

$\Delta\%PV = 100\times[(Hb_{pre}/Hb_{post})\times(1-Hct_{post}/1-Hct_{pre})]$

Figure 13. Baseline blood measurement, being taken prior to the start of the TAC 2004 at Mittenwald/BRD.

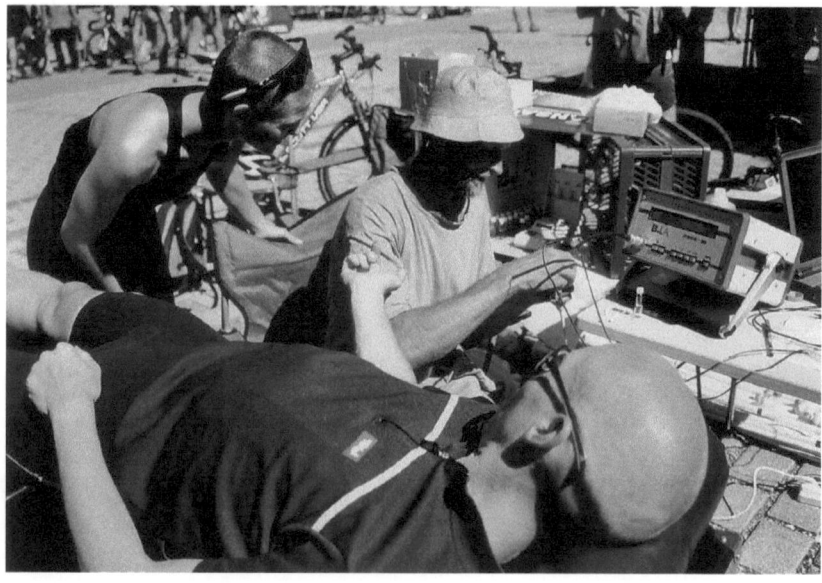

2.4.5. Vegan nutrition pattern

Specific recommendations for fluid intake were adopted from Maughan (2002) and Jeukendrup (2002a). Current recommendations for carbohydrate (CHO) intake were adopted (Burke 2002, Hargreaves 2002, Jentjens 2002, Jeukendrup 2002a). Using a self-reported 24 hour survey, the dietary intake was completely recorded over the full period of eight successive days of competition with the maximum possible accuracy. Fluid intake (FI) and energy intake (EI) were calculated for three time periods and subdivided into macronutrients CHO, protein and fat:
1) Pre race (breakfast)
2) Race (sports drink, solid energy bars and energy gels)
3) Post race (including snacks and dinner)

The full period of 24 hours was accounted for by pre race period (6 – 8 a. m.), daily runtime, time for sleep (10 p. m. – 6 a. m.) and post exercise recovery period, which was found on average to be 8 hours 45 minutes.

The recorded daily FI took into consideration the kind of fluid and was calculated from both the reported number and content of ingested cups, glasses and bottles of fluid and drinking bottles of sport drinks down to an accuracy of 125 mL. The energy value and contents of ingested sport drinks of prepared and packed commercial substrate was available from their food labels. Furthermore, the energy value and nutritional data of any alcohol consumed was derived from producer's declarations, obtained by contacting the producers following personal conversations with the head waiter.

The energy content and composition of prepared and packed commercial energy food (solid bars and gels) were taken from the manufacturer's declaration. The energy content and detailed information for pieced and/or portioned food (such as bread, pate, fresh or dried fruit, snacks) were taken directly from food labels, where available. Otherwise, the mass of pieces and/or portions of food was weighed using kitchen scales (accuracy of 10 g: Culina Plus, Soehnle, Germany). Based on personal communication with the chef of any bed & breakfast or restaurant, the EI was then calculated from the detailed nutritional information of standardized portions (e. g. type of bread, ingredients, distribution of macronutrients). Similarly, the analysis and calculation of EI of a specific dish of combined food (such as standardized portions of pizza and pasta,) was derived from nutritional data (as described above) after personal conversation with the relevant cook. From this information, if no food label or further description of nutritional content from other sources was available (which could be totalled to a negligible magnitude), the calculation of total EI and the respective macronutrients for each piece, portion or combined dish of food was determined by using the nutritional information chart of Petter and Pohlmann (2007) as well as some standardized food composition databases available online (www.bleibfit.at, www.dge.de, www.naehrwerttabelle.de).

The translation of units was calculated according to the Systeme International d' Unites (SI: www.bipm.org, www.bipm.org/en/CGPM/db/11/12/). Following this concept, the energy of 1 kcal equates to 4.1868 kJ (http://ester.chemie.fu-berlin.de/cgi-bin/units?from=kcal&to=kJ&have=&want). The quantity of energy ingested was calculated according to Geiss and Hamm (1992): 1 gram of CHO equates to 4.1 kcal, 1 gram of protein to 4.1 kcal and 1 gram of fat to 9.3 kcal.

2.5. Statistical analysis

Descriptive data are presented as mean ± standard deviation (SD). After performing the Shapiro–Wilk test, the data was found to be normal distributed. Due to the small sample sizes, non–parametric tests were used for all the analyses.

The differences in average values of RPE, exercise induced FI, HR between the eight stages, and the differences in the time spent within each of the four intensity zones during each stage were examined using the Friedman test and Wilcoxon paired tests as post–hoc analyses. Likewise, the differences in average values of body water compartments between baseline and Stage 1, Stage 1 and 4, and between Stage 1 and 6, were examined using the Friedman test and Wilcoxon paired tests (post–hoc). Analyses were performed by using SPSS software package (version 15.0, Chicago, Illinois, USA). The level of statistical significance was set at p≤0.05.

Haematological parameters were analyzed by using SPSS software package, version 11.0 (Chicago, Illinois, USA). Changes in average values of Hb, Hct and PV_{CALC} were examined by paired t test as post–hoc analyses. Correlations were calculated using Pearson`s correlation coefficient (r).

3. Results

The athletes had to cope with high temperatures for almost two third of the whole race (28 – 33 °C) with an average temperature of 28 °C. Six of the eight stages were competed under dry conditions (44 – 50 % relative humidity).

3.1. Questionnaire

The results of the questionnaire evaluation are shown in Figure 14 and Table 5. After the rating of MTBers the TAC 2004 was perceived overall to be "hard (heavy)". Additionally, fatigue of leg muscles was reported to be "okay", confirming the RPE results (15.2 points). Furthermore, mood situation was rated to be "good" during the whole period of TAC 2004. Average of daily FI consumed from breakfast to finish of stage was 4.5 L.

Figure 14. Temperature (T), relative humidity (rh), exercise induced fluid intake since breakfast (FI) and rate of perceived exertion (RPE) during the Transalp Challenge 2004 are depicted as mean values.

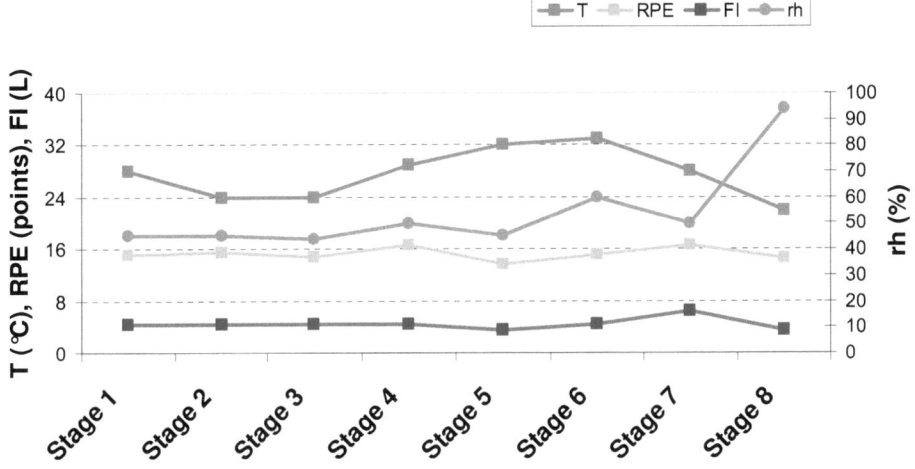

Table 5. Evaluation of questionnaire. Values are mean ± standard deviation (SD). Significant differences compared to Stage 1 are defined as follows: ** ($p \leq 0.01$), * ($p \leq 0.05$). RPE = rate of perceived exertion (Borg 1998). v. g. = very good. g = good, o. k. = okay.

	Unit	Stage 1	Stage 2	Stage 3	Stage 4	Stage 5	Stage 6	Stage 7	Stage 8	Mean (±SD)	Range
Number		30	29	24	25	23	21	13	11	22 (±7)	11 – 30
Parameters											
RPE (6–20)	points	15.1 (±1.9)	15.4 (±1.9)	14.8 (±1.5)	16.5 (±1.9)**	13.7 (±2.3)	15.1 (±1.8)	16.6 (±2.4)**	14.6 (±2.7)	15.2 (±1.0)	9 – 20
Fluid intake	L	4.4 (±1.0)	4.5 (±1.3)	4.4 (±1.3)	4.6 (±0.9)	3.5 (±1.0)*	4.5 (±1.6)	6.4 (±1.2)*	3.3 (±1.3)**	4.5 (±0.9)	2 – 10
Mood	Smilie	v. g./good	v. g./good	v. g./good	good/o. k.	v. g./good	v. g./good	good	v. g./good	Good ☺	v. g/o. k.
Muscles of legs	Smilie	o. k.	o. k.	o. k.	o. k.	o. k.	o. k.	o. k.	o. k./bad	o. k. ☺	o. k./bad

3.2. Exercise intensity

The characteristics of subjects are shown in Table 6.

Table 6. Physiological characteristics of riders and results of incremental laboratory test (starting at 100 W, steps of 30 W every 5 min) are mean ± SD. HR = heart rate, PO = power output, PPO = peak PO, LT = fixed lactate threshold of 2 (LT2), 4 (LT4) and 6 (LT6) mmol/L, bpm = beats/minute.

	Unit	Male (n=5)	Female (n=2)	Pooled (n=7)
Age	years	33.6 (±3.0)	34.7 (±3.0)	32.0 (±3.0)
Body mass	kg	63.3 (±10.0)	51.0 (±1.4)	58.4 (±10.0)
Height	cm	1.71 (±0.4)	1.63 (±2.1)	1.67 (±5.4)
Absolute PPO	W	314 (±43)	242 (±40)	285 (±54)
	W/kg	4.8 (±0.3)	4.1 (±0.6)	4.5 (±0.5)
PO at LT2	W	202 (±11)	189 (±22)	197 (±15)
	W/kg	3.3 (±0.6)	3.2 (±0.5)	3.2 (±0.5)
PO at LT4	W	249 (±12)	214 (±21)	235 (±23)
	W/kg	4.0 (±0.6)	3.6 (±0.6)	3.8 (±0.6)
PO at LT6	W	273 (±22)	228 (±21)	255 (±31)
	W/kg	4.4 (±0.5)	3.8 (±0.6)	4.1 (±0.5)
Maximal HR	bpm	174 (±2)	183 (±0.7)	177 (±5)
HR at LT2	bpm	140 (±16)	155 (±1)	146 (±14)
	% max	80.4 (±9.5)	84.4 (±0.3)	82.0 (±7.0)
HR at LT4	bpm	157 (±4)	168 (±3)	161 (±7)
	% max	90.2 (±2.6)	92.1 (±1.2)	91.0 (±2.2)
HR at LT6	bpm	166 (±3)	173 (± 7)	169 (±6)
	% max	95.6 (±2.3)	94.8 (±3.5)	95.3 (±2.4)

The findings of exercise intensity during the course of the TAC 2004 are presented in Tables 7 and 10 (case study). The average exercise intensity of 85 % of maximum HR during racing was maintained over the full period of eight successive stages of TAC 2004. As a consequence, the average HR expressed as percentage of $HR_{MAX}Lab$ was lower than that expressed as percentage of $HR_{MAX}Field$ from stage 2 to 8 ($p<0.05$). The decline in absolute maximal HR was significant ($p<0.05$) with differences found between Stage 1 and stages 2 to 8.

The exercise intensity indicated by mean RPE was determined to be 16.1 points with significant differences found between Stage 1 and stages 2 (+1.8 points, p=0.02), 4 (+1.2 points, p=0.05), 5 (−2.8 points, p=0.05) and 7 (+2.6 points, p=0.02).

Relative FI was 10 ± 10 mL/kg*h while racing. Body mass remained stable throughout the stage race (pooled data pre race: 58.4 ± 9.9 kg, pooled data post race: 58.6 ± 9.9 kg).

Table 7. Pooled data (n=7) of exercise intensity (HR = heart rate, RPE = rate of perceived exertion) during the Transalp Challenge 2004 are presented as mean ± standard deviation (SD). Significant differences compared to Stage 1 are defined as follows: *(p≤0.02), °(p=0.03), □(p≤0.05). HRave = average HR, HR$_{MAX}$ = maximal HR, %HR$_{MAX}$Field = values of HR expressed as percentage of maximal HR during race, %HR$_{MAX}$Lab = values of HR expressed as percentage of maximal HR during laboratory testing. FI = race induced fluid intake since breakfast, bpm = beats/min.

	Unit	Stage 1	Stage 2	Stage 3	Stage 4	Stage 5	Stage 6	Stage 7	Stage 8	Mean (±SD)
Stage time	min	307	349	286	415	279	289	443	289	326 (±61)
HRave	bpm	149 (±11)	138 (±6)	142 (±2)	141 (±2)	140 (±5)	139 (±3)	139 (±3)	137 (±3)	141 (±5)
HRave	%HR$_{MAX}$Field	85 (±5)	83 (±4)	85 (±2)	87 (±2)	87 (±2)	84 (±3)	87 (±2)	86 (±3)	85 (±2)
HRave	%HR$_{MAX}$Lab	84 (±6)	78 (±3)*	80 (±1)	80 (±1)*	79 (±3)*	76 (±4)*	78 (±2)*	78 (±2)*	79 (±1)
HR$_{MAX}$	bpm	176 (±6)	166 (±5)*	167 (±3)°	162 (±4)*	162 (±3)*	165 (±6)*	160 (±2)*	161 (±6)*	165 (±4)
HR$_{MAX}$	%HR$_{MAX}$Lab	99 (±3)	94 (±3)	94 (±2)°	91 (±3)	91 (±2)	93 (±3)	90 (±1)	91 (±3)	93 (±2)
Uphill cycling										
HRave	bpm	154 (±13)	143 (±7)*	142 (±5)°	144 (±4)	149 (±3)	145 (±4)	141 (±3)	143 (±6)	146 (±6)
HRave	%HR$_{MAX}$Field	87 (±5)	86 (±4)	85 (±4)	89 (±3)	92 (±1)	88 (±3)	89 (±1)	89 (±5)	88 (±2)
HR$_{MAX}$	bpm	170 (±7)	158 (±5)*	159 (±5)□	155 (±5)*	161 (±3)°	162 (±4)	156 (±3)*	153 (±5)*	160 (±5)
HR$_{MAX}$	%HR$_{MAX}$Field	97 (±3)	95 (±2)	96 (±1)	96 (±2)	≤100 (±0)	98 (±2)	98 (±1)	94 (±4)	97 (±1)
Downhill cycling										
HRave	bpm	138 (±11)	125 (±5)*	123 (±8)*	129 (±4)□	130 (±3)	137 (±4)	124 (±2)*	120 (±4)°	129 (±5)
HRave	%HR$_{MAX}$Field	79 (±5)	75 (±3)*	74 (±5)*	80 (±3)	80 (±1)	83 (±2)	78 (±1)*	75 (±4)*	78 (±2)
HR$_{MAX}$	bpm	160 (±8)	148 (±6)*	146 (±7)*	151 (±6)*	153 (±4)	159 (±6)	144 (±4)*	142 (±5)*	151 (±6)
HR$_{MAX}$	%HR$_{MAX}$Field	91 (±4)	89 (±4)	87 (±5)	93 (±3)	94 (±1)	96 (±2)	90 (±2)	88 (±4)	91 (±2)
RPE (6–20)	points	15.4 (±0.9)	17.2 (±1.1)*	16.6 (±2.5)	16.6 (±1.8)□	12.6 (±2.6)□	16.4 (1.3)	18.0 (±1.0)*	15.8 (±2.2)	16.1 (±0.5)
FI	L	4.4 (±1.1)	4.2 (±1.5)	3.7 (±1.4)	4.4 (±1.4)	3.2 (±1.2)°	3.8 (±1.5)	5.3 (±1.5)	2.8 (±1.2)□	4.2 (±1.1)

Figure 15 depicts the distribution of time spent in respective intensity zones. Values were analyzed independent of gender due to the lack of significance in results of absolute and relative HR between sexes. The distribution of exercise intensity during the 8 stages, expressed as percentage of $HR_{MAX}Field$ and $HR_{MAX}Lab$, is shown in Figure 16. The mean time expressed as percentage of total race time in the low, moderate, high and very high–intensity zones was determined using the $HR_{MAX}Lab$ were 36 ± 12 %, 58 ± 13%, 4 ± 8 % and 2 ± 9 %, respectively (Figure 16A). When the intensity zones were determined using the $HR_{MAX}Field$ the time spent in the low, moderate, high and very high–intensity zones was 23 ± 8 %, 41 ± 14 %, 27 ± 14 % and 9 ± 9 % of total race time (Figure 16C). The percentage of the total race time spent in the intensity zones as determined with $HR_{MAX}Field$ was different from the time spent in the intensity zones calculated using the $HR_{MAX}Lab$ (Figure 16B).

Figure 15. Time spent in respective intensity zones LOW, MODERATE, HIGH and VERY HIGH as determined by %$HR_{MAX}Field$ (n=7) during the Transalp Challenge 2004. Values are means ± SD.

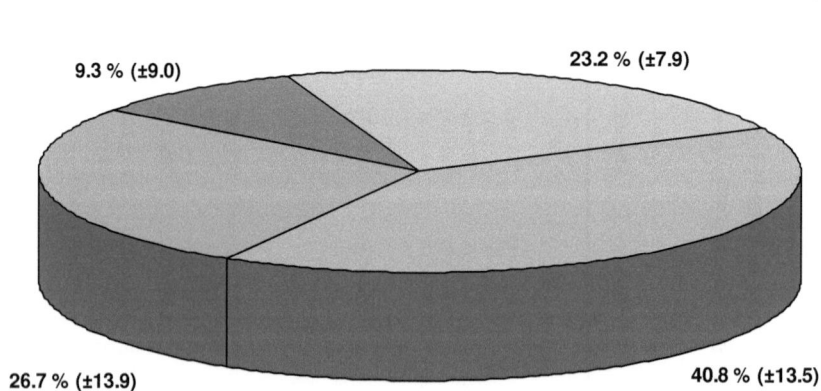

Figure 16. Percentage of total stage time daily spent in respective intensity zones LOW, MODERATE, HIGH and VERY HIGH. MOD = MODERATE zone. Each bar in respective load zone corresponds to stages 1 to 8 in natural order. Figures 16A and 16C indicate differences (based on absolute HR) from Stage 1. Figure 16B depicts the differences in the total stage time (based on $HR_{MAX}Lab$ versus $HR_{MAX}Field$) for each single stage 1 to 8. Significant differences: *($p<0.05$)

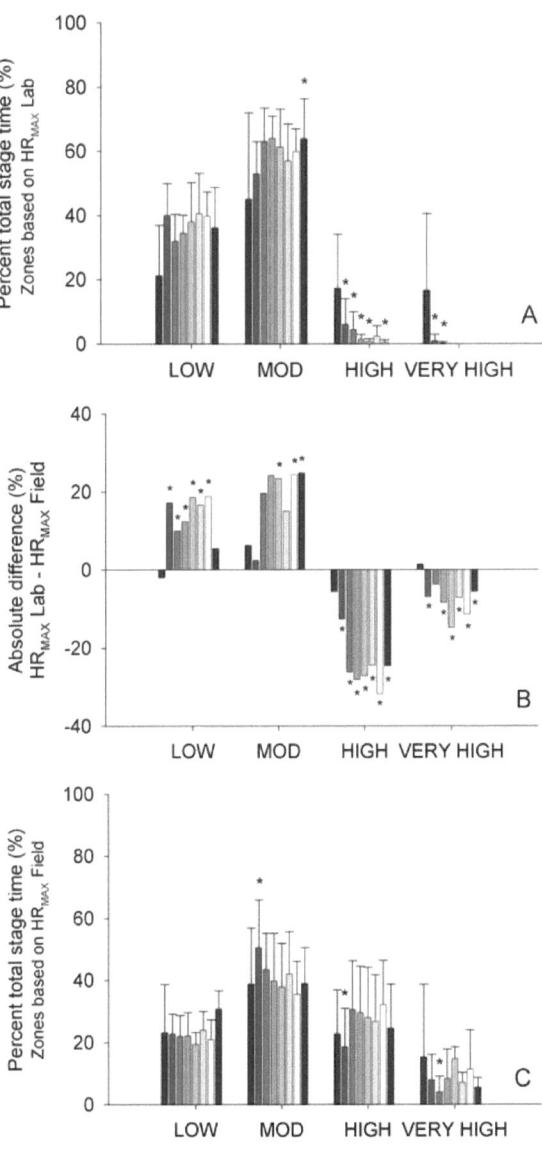

3.3. Status of body water and haematology

Values of body water pools and haematological parameters are presented as pooled data due to the lack of significance between sexes (Table 8). Relative FI had an average of 10 ± 10 mL/kg*h for both study groups during daily race.

Compared to euhydrated adults (De Marees 2003), baseline data of extracellular water (ECW) are shown to be considerably enhanced for mean values (+24.1 %), whereas data of baseline intracellular water (ICW) show a pronounced decline at the same time (–10.0 %). Acute changes after first stage of TAC 2004 show a fall in total body water (TBW), ECW and ICW of –2.8 %, –4.1 % and –1.6 %, respectively. Long term adaptations during the TAC 2004 are demonstrated by increased body water pools (Stage 1 to 4: TBW: +7.5 %, ECW: +11.5 %, ICW: +4.5 % and Stage 1 to 6: TBW: +12.6 %, ECW: +19.3 %, ICW: +7.7 %).

The results of haematological parameters are further shown in Figure 17. During the first stage of the TAC 2004 a considerable decline in calculated PV was detected. Simultaneously, a rise in Hb (+17.2 %) and Hct was found. In the course of the TAC 2004 PV was calculated to have expanded, while levels of both Hb (Stage 1 to 4: –19.5 %, Stage 1 to 6: –23.1 %) and Hct fell significantly.

Figure 17. Mean values of hemoglobin (Hb), hematocrit (Hct) and calculated plasma volume (PV_{CALC}) during the TAC 2004.

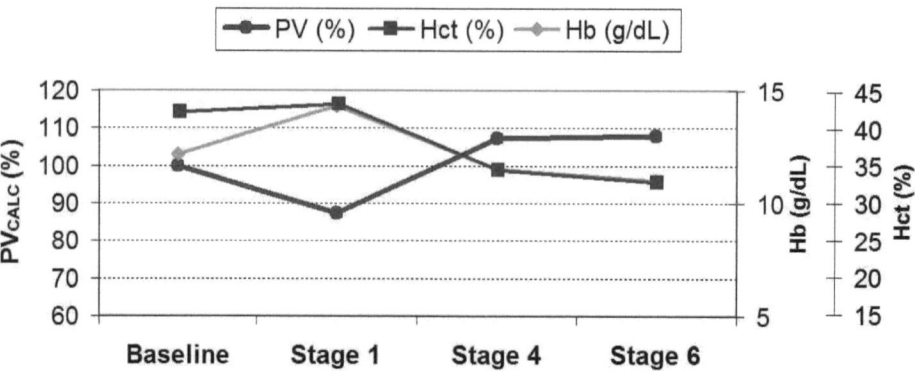

Table 8. Differences in body water status (n=13) and haematological status (n=6) are respectively shown between Baseline and Stage 1 (acute shifts), both Baseline/Stage 1 and Stage 4, and both Baseline/Stage 1 and Stage 6 (long term effects). Values are mean ± standard deviation (SD). Significant differences are defined as follows: ** ($p \leq 0.01$), * ($p \leq 0.05$). TBW = total body water, ECW = extracellular water, ICW = intracellular water. FI = Fluid intake reported from breakfast to daily finish. Hb = hemoglobin, Hct = hematocrit, PV_{CALC} = calculated plasma volume.

	Unit	Baseline	Stage 1	Stage 2	Stage 3	Stage 4	Stage 5	Stage 6	Stage 7	Stage 8
Body water status (n=13)										
TBW	L	42.4 (±6.3)	41.2 (±7.0)	–	–	44.3 (±8.3)	–	46.4 (±8.4)	–	–
ECW	L	17.3 (±2.5)	16.6 (±2.6)	–	–	18.5 (±3.2)	–	19.8 (±3.0)	–	–
ICW	L	25.1 (±3.9)	24.7 (±4.5)	–	–	25.8 (±5.3)	–	26.6 (±5.5)	–	–
Difference TBW	L	–	−1.2 (±1.8)	–	–	+3.1 (±3.9)*	–	+5.2 (±5.5)**	–	–
Difference ECW	L	–	−0.7 (±0.8)**	–	–	+1.9 (±1.5)**	–	+3.2 (±2.3)**	–	–
Difference ICW	L	–	−0.4 (±1.1)	–	–	+1.1 (±2.6)	–	+1.9 (±3.2)*	–	–
FI	L	–	4.4 (±0.9)	–	–	5.0 (±1.3)	–	4.2 (±1.3)	–	–
Haematological status (n=6)										
Hb	g/dL	12.2 (±0.8)	14.3 (±1.8)	–	–	11.5 (±1.8)	–	11.0 (±1.6)	–	–
Hct	%	42.3 (±3.8)	43.2 (±3.4)	–	–	36.8 (±3.1)	–	35.7 (±4.5)	–	–
Difference Hb (to Baseline)	g/dL	–	+2.1 (±1.2)**	–	–	−0.7 (±0.2)	–	−1.2 (±0.6)*	–	–
Difference Hb (to Stage 1)	g/dL	–	–	–	–	−2.8 (±1.6)**	–	−3.3 (±1.9)**	–	–
Difference Hct (to Baseline)	%	–	+0.9 (±1.5)	–	–	−5.5 (±2.3)*	–	−6.6 (±2.8)**	–	–
Difference Hct (to Stage 1)	%	–	–	–	–	−6.4 (±2.7)**	–	−7.5 (±3.2)**	–	–
PV_{CALC}	%	100	87.2 (±6.9)*	–	–	105.5 (±13.1)	–	106.9 (±14.3)	–	–
Difference PV_{CALC} (to Baseline)	%	–	−12.8 (±6.9)*	–	–	+5.5 (±13.1)	–	+6.9 (±14.3)	–	–
Difference PV_{CALC} (to Stage 1)	%	–	–	–	–	+18.3 (±14.9)	–	+19.7 (±15.1)	–	–
FI	L	–	4.3 (±0.9)	–	–	4.8 (±1.2)	–	4.3 (±1.4)	–	–

The haematological ranges representing 95 % of normal population (Eichner 1992): Hb_{men}: 13.3 – 17.7 g/dL, Hct_{men}: 35 – 52 %
The cut off limits for Hb accepted by the FIS (Federation Internationale de Ski; Schumacher et. al. 2000): Hb_{men} > 18.5 g/dL and Hb_{women} > 16.5 g/dL
The cut off limits for Hct accepted by the UCI (Schumacher et. al. 2000): Hct_{men} > 50 % and Hct_{women} > 47 %

3.4. Vegan nutrition pattern

The characteristics of female vegan MTBer is shown in Table 9.

The female vegan MTBer finished the TAC 2004 in 41 hours 59 minutes 45 seconds, overall achieving 16th place overall within the "Mixed" category (with the world elite of professional XC and XCM athletes on occupying the higher rankings).
The findings of exercise intensity during the TAC 2004 are presented in Table 10. The average daily runtime was 5 hours 15 minutes (ranging between 4 – 7 hours) with an average speed of 15.6 km/h. She maintained an average exercise intensity of 88 % of HR_{MAX}Field during eight days of successive race during the TAC 2004. The distribution of time spent in respective intensity zones is presented in Figure 18.

Table 9. Characteristics of the female vegan MTBer and results of incremental laboratory test seven days before the start of the Transalp Challenge 2004 (starting at 100 W, steps of 30 W every 5 min). HR = heart rate, PO = power output, PPO = peak PO, LT = fixed lactate threshold of 2 (LT2), 4 (LT4) and 6 (LT6) mmol/L, bpm = beats/minute.

	Unit	Female MTBer
Anthropological characteristics		
Age	years	30
Body mass (nude)	kg	47
Body mass	kg	50
Height	cm	161
Body mass Index (nude)	–	17.5
Haematological characteristics		
Iron	µg/dL	105
Transferrin	mg/dL	238
Transferrin saturation	%	31
Hemoglobin	g/dL	14
Hematocrit	%	41
Vitamin B12	pg/mL	280
Physiological Characteristics		
Absolute PPO	W	230
	W/kg	4.6
PO at LT2	W	174
	W/kg	3.5
	% max	76.1
PO at LT4	W	199
	W/kg	4.0
	% max	87.0
PO at LT6	W	213
	W/kg	4.3
	% max	93.5
Maximal HR	bpm	182
HR at LT2	bpm	154
	% max	84.6
HR at LT4	bpm	166
	% max	91.2
HR at LT6	bpm	168
	% max	92.3

Table 10. Exercise intensity (HR = heart rate, RPE = rate of perceived exertion) of female vegan MTBer during the Transalp Challenge 2004 are presented as mean ± standard deviation (SD). HRave = average HR, HR_{MAX} = maximal HR, $\%HR_{MAX}$Field = values of HR expressed as percentage of maximal HR during race, $\%HR_{MAX}$Lab = values of HR expressed as percentage of maximal HR during laboratory testing, bpm = beats/minute.

	Unit	Stage 1	Stage 2	Stage 3	Stage 4	Stage 5	Stage 6	Stage 7	Stage 8	Mean (±SD)
Stage time	min	293	328	287	402	225	280	426	278	315 (±60)
Speed	km/h	16.4	13.4	15.5	17.8	14.4	15.6	17.5	14.5	15.6 (±1.5)
HRave	bpm	164	142	142	143	143	140	138	132	143 (±9)
HRave	$\%HR_{MAX}$Field	91	87	87	88	88	86	87	86	88 (±2)
HRave	$\%HR_{MAX}$Lab	90	78	78	79	79	77	76	73	79 (±5)
HR_{MAX}	bpm	181	164	164	162	163	162	158	154	164 (±8)
HR_{MAX}	$\%HR_{MAX}$Lab	99	90	90	89	90	89	87	85	90 (±4)
Uphill cycling										
Time	min	228	252	210	220	150	197	233	179	209 (±33)
Speed	km/h	11.5	10.5	11.3	12.6	9.2	10.6	17.8	4.9	11.1 (±3.6)
Downhill cycling										
Time	min	60	61	63	110	75	83	79	88	77 (±17)
Speed	km/h	29.1	26.0	25.5	36.6	22.0	25.0	21.4	23.8	26.2 (±4.9)
RPE (6–20)	points	15	17	19	14	15	17	17	18	16.5 (±1.7)

Figure 18. Time spent by female vegan rider in respective intensity zones LOW, MODERATE, HIGH and VERY HIGH as determined by %HR_{MAX}Field during the Transalp Challenge 2004.

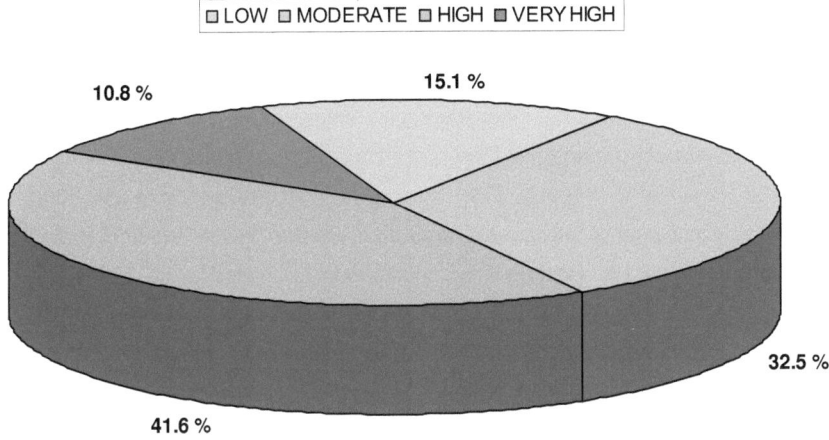

Dietary intake. Tables 11 – 13 and Figure 19 depict the dietary intake during the whole period of TAC 2004. The average EI was found to be 24.61 MJ/day. During the TAC 2004, dietary intake reached maximum values with a FI of 4.5 L and an EI of 3116 kcal during "king size" Stage 7. In contrast, values were minimal during the cool and rainy Stage 8 (FI was 1.5 L, EI was 1409 kcal).

Fluid intake. Daily FI ranged from 4.25 L to 7.75 L, reflecting a daily average of 5.48 L. Fluid ingested during breakfast, averaging of 200 mL/day (3.7 % of total FI), came exclusively from tea (English or Green) without sugar. The fluid ingested while racing came exclusively from isotonic sport drinks rich in CHO, accounting for 24 L (3 L/stage). This volume amounts to 54.7 % of the total FI ingested during the whole TAC 2004. Expressed as relative terms, the female consumed 12 mL/kg*h during racing, which is 570 mL/h runtime. The MTBer ingested 59 g of CHO/L during racing (6 % solution). The total energy consumed exclusively from sport drinks was 20.1 MJ, reflecting 30.6 % of CHO intake during daily racing. Furthermore, 12.3 % of the total CHO intake during the entire TAC 2004 came from CHO consumed with isotonic sport drinks. FI during post race period came exclusively from water (tap, table and mineral) accounting for 17.1 L. Alcoholic drinks, solely consumed after the finish of TAC 2004, accounted for 1.125 L. Together, post exercise FI derived from water and alcohol contributed 41.6 % of total FI.

Energy and macronutrient intake. The EI broken down by time periods is presented in Table 12. The most important occasions to eat were post race, accounting for 47.4 % of total EI. The EI during daily racing was found to be 94.9 % derived from CHO, reflecting 40.1 % of total CHO intake during the entire TAC 2004. Similarly, 44.2 % of total CHO intake was consumed during the post race period while breakfast only accounted for a smaller amount of 15.7 % of total CHO intake during the full period of TAC 2004.

The distribution of total calories was 83.3 % from CHO, 7.5 % from protein and 9.2 % from fat (Figure 19). Relative CHO intake was calculated to be 24.4 g/kg*day (100 kcal/kg*day). An average of 188 g CHO (3.8 g CHO/kg) was ingested daily during breakfast. The relative amounts of CHO ingested daily during racing were 9.8 g CHO/kg body mass and 91.2 g CHO/h runtime. Relative CHO intake during daily racing was calculated to be 32 kJ/kg*h (7.63 kcal/kg*h). Relative daily post race ingestion from CHO was 1.2 g/kg*h (60.4 g CHO/h). Daily amounts consumed of fat and protein consumed totalled 58 g/day (1.2 g/kg*day) and 107 g/day (2.2 g/kg*day), respectively.

Food groups. EI from the most important food groups are shown in Table 13. During the TAC 2004, the most important food groups were found to be energy food (solid energy bars, gels, drinks) which accounted for 35.2 % of total EI consumed.

Energy exclusively from solid energy bars and gels accounted for 49.1 MJ (6.1 MJ/day). Taken together, 25 % of total EI during the whole period of TAC 2004 came from solid energy food. The main source of CHO, besides energy food, was bread, (26.9 %) as well as pizza and pasta. Calories from fruit was calculated to be 4.3 %, including 2.8 % of total EI (5.56 MJ) coming from bananas.

Table 11. Energy intake (EI) and fluid intake (FI) of female vegan MTBer for each time period during the Transalp Challenge 2004.

	Unit	Stage 1	Stage 2	Stage 3	Stage 4	Stage 5	Stage 6	Stage 7	Stage 8	Total	Mean (±SD)
Breakfast											
EI	kcal	1512.5	983.2	804.6	1782	737.4	782.5	491.6	1085.6	8179	1022 (±429)
FI	L	0.125	0.25	0.25	0.25	0.25	0.125	0.25	0.125	1.625	0.20 (±0.06)
Race											
EI	kcal	1929.6	2151.6	2373.6	1930	1930	1711	3116	1408.8	16550	2069 (±510)
FI	L	3	3	3	3	3	3	4.5	1.5	24	3 (±0.8)
Post Race											
EI	kcal	2594.8	2536.4	1586.8	1309	3192	2943	3844	4024.1	22300	2787 (±925)
FI	L	1.8	1.8	1.0	1.5	3.0	2.5	3.0	3.63	18.23	2.28 (±0.9)
Total TAC 2004											
EI	kcal	6036.9	5671.2	5035	5021	5859.4	5436.5	7451.6	6518.5	47030	5878 (±810)
	MJ	25.28	23.74	21.08	21.02	24.53	22.76	31.2	27.29	196.91	24.61 (±3.39)
FI	L	4.93	5.05	4.25	4.75	6.25	5.63	7.75	5.25	43.85	5.48 (±1.1)
Body mass	kg	48	50	48	49	50	50	50	50	–	49 (±1)

Figure 19. Macronutrient contribution for each time period and whole Transalp Challenge 2004. CHO = carbohydrate.

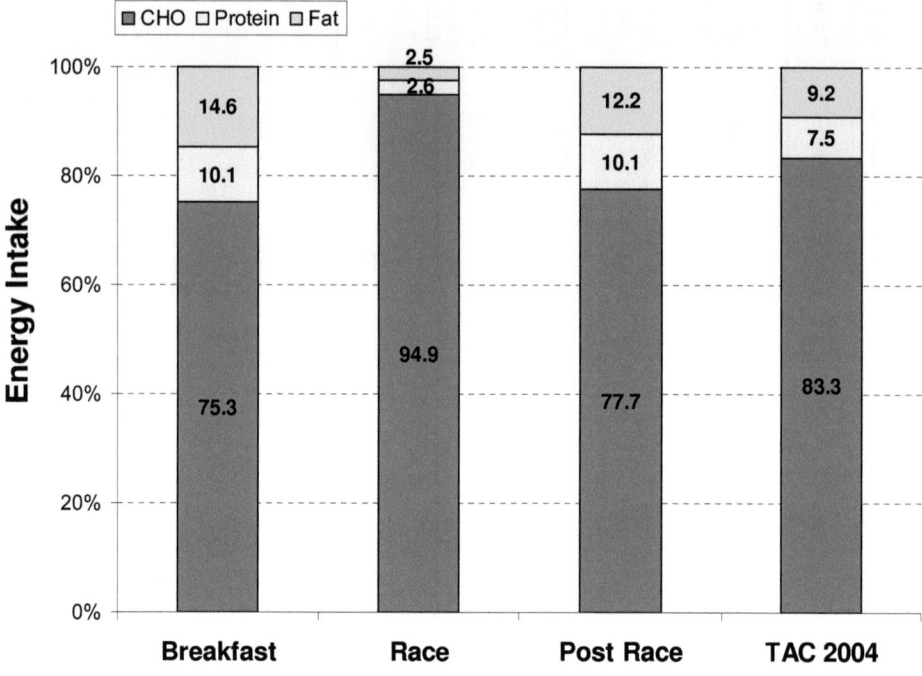

Table 12. Distribution of macronutrients carbohydrate (CHO), protein and fat for each time period. g = gram, kcal = kilocalorie, kJ = kilojoule, MJ = megajoule.

	g	kcal	kJ	MJ	% Dish	% Total
Breakfast	1831	8180	34246	34.24		17.40 %
CHO	1501	6156	25774	25.77	75.30 %	
Protein	202	830	3474	3.47	10.10 %	
Fat	128	1194	4998	5	14.60 %	
Race	3980	16550	69293	69.30		35.20 %
CHO	3831	15706	65757	65.76	94.90 %	
Protein	104	426	1785	1.79	2.60 %	
Fat	45	418	1751	1.75	2.50 %	
Post Race	5069	22301	93370	93.37		47.40 %
CHO	4228	17334	72574	72.57	77.70 %	
Protein	548	2247	9407	9.41	10.10 %	
Fat	293	2720	11389	11.39	12.20 %	
Total TAC 2004	10880	47030	196909	196.91		
CHO	9560	39196	164105	164.11		83.30 %
Protein	854	3503	14666	14.67		7.50 %
Fat	466	4332	18138	18.14		9.20 %

Table 13. Distribution of energy intake from the most important vegan food groups during the whole period of Transalp Challenge 2004. kcal = kilocalorie, kJ = kilojoule, MJ = megajoule.

	kcal	kJ	MJ	% Total EI	% Total EI
Energy food			69.29		35.20 %
Bars	3285	13754		7.0 %	
Gels	8436	35320		17.94 %	
Drinks	4829	20128		10.22 %	
Combined food			34.62		17.60 %
Pizza	2318	9704		4.93 %	
Pasta	5950	24912		12.65 %	
Snacks & others			84.39		42.90 %
Potatoes	243	1015		0.52 %	
Bread	12640	52921		26.88 %	
Fruit (incl. banana)	2016	8441		4.29 %	
Sweets	2886	12083		6.14 %	
Marmelade & Pate	577	2414		1.23 %	
Cereals	1795	7515		3.82 %	

4. Discussion

The focus of this chapter is mainly on the most important factors that might determine, or rather limit, MTB performance during competition in the TAC. The requirements an athlete has to face when participating in the TAC are highlighted by a complex performance capacity, amongst others, including the following aspects:

4.1. Physiological parameters

4.1.1. Physiological profile of the MTB athlete

Regarding performance determining factors and physiological profile in MTB sports (Impellizzeri et. al. 2002/2005a+b, Lee et. al. 2002, Stapelfeldt et al. 2004, Wilber et. al. 1997), a completely different profile of skills and physiological characteristics of the MTB athlete was found in comparison to road cycling. These are due to an enormous peak PO, particularly at the beginning of a race, and a permanent change of load and recovery during the whole event. The individual performance during MTB races is characterized by very high intensities and a very high impact distribution during the whole competition (Impellizzeri et. al. 2002/2005a+b, Stapelfeldt et. al. 2004: 88 – 93 % HR_{MAX} in XC; Wirnitzer and Kornexl 2008, Wirnitzer 2009a+b: 85 – 88 % HR_{MAX} in TAC 2004).

On the one hand, the importance of single skills for the MTB performance markedly differs from those for road cycling. On the other hand, the physiologic–anthropometrical characteristics of MTBers are very similar to those of road cycling uphill specialists (Impellizzeri et. al. 2002, Lee et. al. 2002, Prins et. al. 2007, Wilber et. al. 1997). MTBers show a higher relative PPO (W/kg) at maximum load. For example Karl Platt (Germany), professional MTB athlete and 7 times winner of the TAC, showed absolute and relative data (maximal aerobic incremental test in spring 2007) of peak PO to be 410 W and 5.86 W/kg (Scheele and Grieshaber 2007). Stapelfeldt et. al. (2004) reported a relative peak PO of 4.5 W/kg in one female elite MTBer of the German national team (age: 30 years, height: 1.70 m, body mass: 62 kg). From personal communication with coaches of national and international MTB team members as well as multiple time winners of UCI XCM races and winners and runners–up of the overall XCM WC, the bench mark for obtaining professional status in female MTB sports might be given as 4.5 W/kg, for obtaining womens world elite in MTB sports a range of 4.7 – 5.0 W/kg might be stated, respectively. However, the female vegan athlete (relative peak PO: 4.6 W/kg) could be classified as a very well endurance trained non–professional MTBer.

Success in MTB sports is basically founded on a high power–to–weight ratio (Lee et. al. 2002). Therefore, training programs should target the improval of relative physiological characteristics rather than the maximization of absolute characteristics to enhance MTB performance (Gregory et. al. 2007, Impellizzeri et. al. 2005a+b, Impellizzeri and Marcora 2007).

4.1.2. Exercise Intensity

Generally, the exercise intensity during mass start stages of a road cycling race, characterized by bunch building and drafting (Figure 20), is clearly lower (Palmer et. al. 1994: 78 – 82 % HR_{MAX}) than during MTB races, in particular for the great 3 Tours (daily runtime of 4 – 7 h over 2 – 3 weeks) ranging from 51 – 65 % HR_{MAX} (Padilla et. al. 2001, Saris et. al. 1989). Mean exercise intensity during the Tour de France was shown to be 60 – 65 % HR_{MAX} (range: 40 – 80 % HR_{MAX}) in two cyclists by HR measurements (Saris et. al. 1989).

Bunch building and drafting is common within mass start road cycle races, as show in Figure 20, taken from Eurosport's live television broadcasting and news programming in cooperation with GETTY IMAGES during the Tour Paris–Nice 2009. Eurosport broadcasts all major cycling races live on a pan–euorpean level. Figure 21 presents an overview of the exercise intensity in MTB sports as compared to road cycling.

Figure 20. Bunch building and drafting during the Tour Paris–Nice 2009 (with permission from 12th August 2009, © Eurosport in cooperation with GETTY IMAGES).

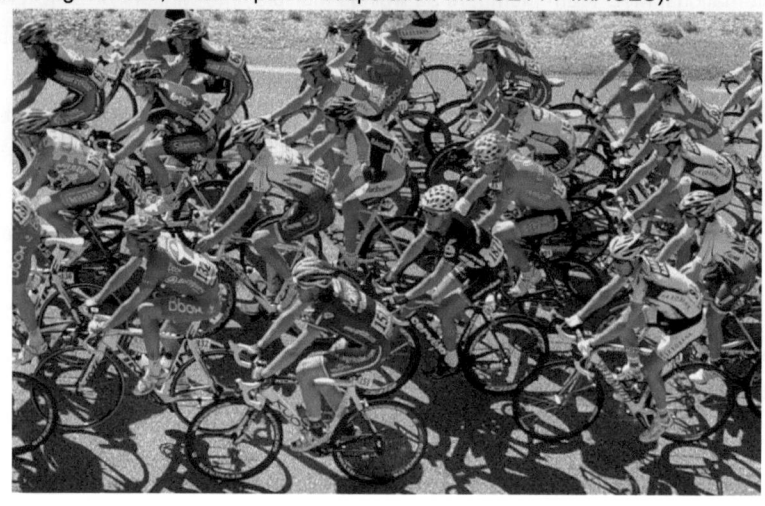

Figure 21. Exercise intensity in MTB sports (single performance) compared to road cycling (single performance, mass start races with bunch building, the great 3 Tours) as percentage of maximum heart rate (HR). XC = cross–country, TAC = Transalp Challenge. HR_{MAX} = maximum HR, ITT & HIMO = individual time trial & high mountain stages (road cycling races). $_1$(Impellizzeri et. al. 2002/2005a+b, Stapelfeldt et. al. 2004), $_2$(Wirnitzer and Kornexl 2008, Wirnitzer 2009a+b), $_3$(Padilla et. al. 2000, Palmer et. al. 1994), $_4$(Palmer et. al. 1994), $_5$(Saris et. al. 1989), $_6$(Padilla et. al. 2001)

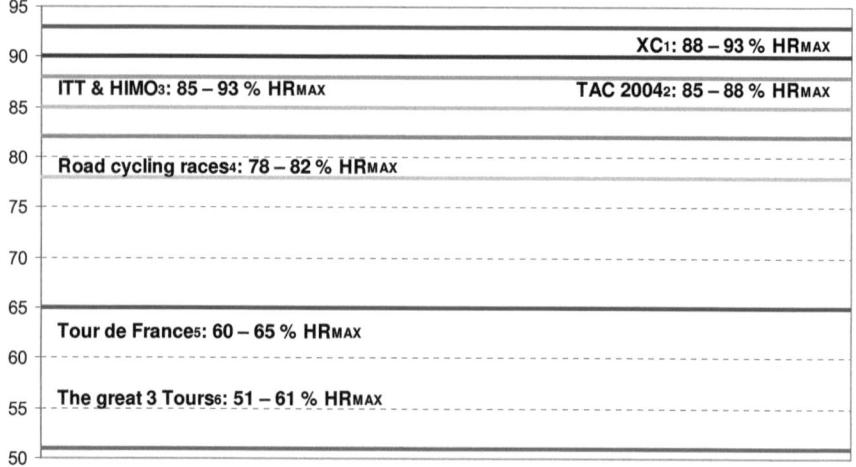

The exercise intensity during Olympic XC races reported in previous studies (Impellizzeri et. al. 2002/2005a+b; Stapelfeldt et. al. 2004) is higher than during the TAC 2004. This can be explained by the shorter duration of Olympic XC (about 2 hours). Most of the studies on road cycling have examined the exercise intensity of the major stage races (Giro d'Italia, Tour de France, Vuelta a Espana). Only two studies have described the exercise intensity of short stage races in professional (Vogt et. al. 2006) and amateur cyclists (Palmer et. al. 1994). Vogt et. al. (2006) showed a mean HR during four stages ranging from 140 – 144 bpm (the HR during the uphill time trial was 169 bpm). Unfortunately they did not report the HR_{MAX} making the comparison with the present findings not possible. On the other hand, Palmer et. al. (1994) showed a mean HR of 82 % and 79 % of the HR_{MAX}Field for the second and fourth stage of a 4–day road race. These figures were similar to the average HRs found during the TAC 2004. However, the stages of the Giro del Capo were only four compared to the eight of the TAC 2004, with the stages 1 and 3 being short time trials (22 and 14 min, respectively). This highlights the high intensity maintained by the MTBers throughout eight days of racing.

The high intensity found during the TAC 2004 can be explained by the characteristics of XC competitions (Impellizzeri et. al. 2002; Impellizzeri and Marcora 2007). Indeed, the XCM as well as the Olympic XC is characterised by a great diversity of terrains and technically very difficult single tracks. Elevated HR in technical elements during downhill sections might be explained due to a high level of concentration and the additional mental stress. This may partially explain the higher mean HR during MTBing compared to on road cycling (further information: Chapter 4.2. Bike handling mastery and race tactics, Chapter 4.4. Mood and mental capacity). Hurst and Atkins (2002/2006) also as Stapelfeldt et. al. (2004) emphasize a paradox for the assessment of downhill performance in MTBing before.

As widely shown in literature, HR data drop as a consequence of repeated bouts of exhaustive exercise during consecutive days, as does impact (high extent and intensity). The diminished decline in HR during road cycling stage races was already reported by Lucia et. al. (2003a) during both Vuelta a Espana (–4.4 % in HR_{MAX}) and Tour de France (–3.9 % in HR_{MAX}) and might be due to race tactics which basically results in a lower average exercise intensity compared to the single performance in MTB. During the Tour de France and Vuelta a Espana Lucia et. al. (2003a) reported a decline of about 0.4 bpm/day corresponding to an 8 bpm decrease after 3–week stage races and about 3 bpm after eight days of racing as in the present report. Fellmann et. al. (1999) found the mean

HR to drop by 9.5 % during a seven–day lasting stage race (453 km on MTB plus running and skiing). Similarly, a fall in mean HR (n=7: –8.1 %; n=1: –19.5 %) and HR_{MAX} (n=7: –8.5 %, n=1: –14.9 %) was shown during the TAC 2004. The maximum HR decreased of 10 bpm (n=7) and 17 bpm (n=1) after Stage 1, but then remained stable. This HR decline was gradual and evident only after the first stage of TAC 2004. As a consequence, the HR expressed as percentage of HR_{MAX}Field did not change significantly throughout the whole stage race.

Mechanisms proposed to explain this HR decline have included catecholamine exhaustion and/or a reduction in sympathetic activity (Lucia et. al. 2003a). Other possible mechanisms can be related to a secondary hypervolemia (further information: Chapter 4.1.3. Body water pools and haematology) occurring as a consequence of acute high intensity exercise in already trained subjects (Richardson et. al. 1996; Wirnitzer and Faulhaber 2007, Wirnitzer and Kornexl 2008, Wirnitzer 2009a+b) or an incomplete restoration of muscle glycogen stores. Especially during stage races, when CHO intake is crucially very high and the next activity starts within the following 8 – 16 hours, glycogen levels will be suboptimal (Jentjens 2002, Jeukendrup 2002a).

Except for secondary hypervolemia or a sparing behaviour during this stage race, neither catecholamine exhaustion nor a reduction in sympathetic activity seem to explain the HR decline found in the TAC 2004. According to the HR response it seems that hydration strategies and CHO replacement have been adequate as shown by a stable body mass in all athletes. An incomplete restoration of glycogen stores might be excluded based on a total recovery time of 16 hours 45 minutes (n=1: post race period and time of sleep). The riders were highly motivated and maintained a very positive mood each to compete and perform at their limit to reach the best final ranking as possible. Moreover, all the riders had experience with the TAC (1 – 6 previous participations). Therefore, sparing behaviour in race tactics might (but ultimately cannot) be excluded. Finally, HR responses are rather not biased by further race tactics (bunch building and/or drafting). Together, the quote of error should be acceptable. Nevertheless, given the difficulty in understanding the origin of this decline (physiological, behavioural or psychological) we presented the exercise intensity using as reference HR the maximum values reached in the laboratory and the field (Tables 7 and 10, Figure 16).

During the TAC, the accumulated total race time spent in HIGH and VERY HIGH intensity zones of 36 % (n=7) and 52.4 % (n=1), respectively related to HR_{MAX}Field, along with the afore mentioned impressive exercise intensity based on HR values, indicate that anaerobic metabolism (the contribution of anaerobic power and capacity to MTB performance) plays a major role in off–road cycling, as formerly suggested in Olympic XC (Baron 2001, Impellizzeri et. al. 2005a+b, Impellizzeri and Marcora 2007, Lee et. al. 2002, Stapelfeldt et. al. 2004). The time spent in LOW and MODERATE intensity zones was 64 % (n=7) and 47.6 % (n=1), respectively as well related to HR_{MAX}Field.

Together, the TAC is currently shown to be physiologically very demanding and heavily involves both the aerobic and anaerobic energy system.

Mean values of overall RPE (16.1 and 16.5 points), corresponding to a perceived effort between "hard (heavy)" and "very hard" (Borg 1998), were found to be highly correlated with mean HR for all stages (n. s.), and with peak temperature and relative humidity during Stage 2 (r=0.92, p=0.01) and Stage 4 (r=0.80, p=0.05). The latter further indicates the high impact of environmental factors on MTB performance (for more detail see Chapter 4.3. Nutritional strategies – Vegan nutrition pattern). Overall, two thirds of RPE is accounted for by physiological factors (central and local) and one third by psychological parameters (Borg 1982/1998/2004). However, overall RPE is highly dependent on the kind of sport (Beneke 1998). Although the trunk musculature is essential for the MTB athlete to stabilize the bike, especially in rough terrain (bike handling), when observing cycling strains, the main muscle groups recruited are leg muscles. It has to be highlighted that fatigue of the muscles of the lower limb, in particular of m. quadriceps, is critical to the MTB performance. Local fatigue of leg muscles considerably influences central and overall fatigue. Therefore, local RPE is strongly related to overall RPE in MTB sports (Garcin et. al. 1998a+b, Jameson and Ring 2000, Johnson et. al. 1985, Koivula and Hassem 1998, Nethery 2002, Robertson et. al. 2000).

The development of TAC in key data and performance over the last decade, indicated as the overall winners` runtime, is displayed in Table 14. Significant differences (p=0.03) between winners` runtimes in different categories (men, masters, mixed, women) were found for every year the TAC has taken place. Differences in total distance, total altitude difference and mean speed were further calculated to be significant (p=0.001) since conducting the first TAC in 1998. Distance was correlated to overall winners time (r=0.78, p=0.003) and total altitude difference (r=0.68, p=0.01). This is nicely illustrated in the years 2002 and 2005. In the TAC 2002, the shortest distance along with the third lowest altitude difference resulted in the fastest total winners` time ever, even hough mean speed was not the highest. Likewise in 2005, the longest total winners` runtime was caused by the combination of the furthest distance the athletes ever had to cope with and the third largest altitude difference since the TAC started.

However, an improvement in performance can be identified in the TAC during the last 10 years. For example, when first TAC is compared to the TAC 2002, the winners finished about 3 hours earlier in 2002 but the small differences in key data (−26.4 km in distance, +1289 m in altitude difference) could not completely explain this improvement. Similarly, considering the relatively constant winners` runtime in 1998, 2000 and 2004 (around 29 h 30 min, within a range of 13 min), the increase in average speed (range: +0.7 km/h to +2.4 km/h) simultaneously with distance (range: +16.2 km to +66.5 km) and altitude difference (range: −170 m to +4206 m), would indicate higher performances.

Factors other than distance, altitude and speed, such as technical developments (diagnosis and training systems (PO, HR) to determine and quantify physiological parameters, frame material, brake and suspension systems), training programs and interventions, nutritional strategies (energy food with high energy density as required in endurance sports) and bike handling ability amongst others, might have influenced this trend of TAC performance within the past decade.

Table 14. Development of key data and overall winners` run time of the Transalp Challenge from 1998 to 2008. Parameters significantly correlated (Pearson`s correlation coefficient) to total distance are defined as follows: °(p=0.003), □(p=0.01).

Transalp Challenge	Distance (km)	Altitude difference□ (m)	Winners time° (h:min:sec)	Speed (km/h)
1998	595.8	18419	29:32:03	20.2
1999	624.0	20325	28:02:39	21.9
2000	646.1	18249	29:33:44	21.9
2001	668.0	22051	32:05:32	20.8
2002	569.4	19708	26:30:28	21.5
2003	651.3	21520	28:45:19	22.6
2004	662.3	22455	29:21:09	22.6
2005	724.4	22293	32:12:38	22.5
2006	665.0	22572	28:51:55	23.0
2007	628.4	20836	27:32:30	22.8
2008	663.6	21623	29:59:26	22.2
Mean (±SD)	645.3 (±41.0)	20914 (±1560)	29:18:51 (±1:43:37)	22.0 (±0.9)

4.1.3. Body water pools and haematology

Changes in body hydration status and haematological parameters are known to considerably influence physical performance, especially in aerobic endurance sports such as road and off–road cycling (Brouns et. al. 1989a+b, Galloway and Maughan 2000, Kleiner 1999, Neumayr et. al. 2002a/2003b, Saris et. al. 1998, Schumacher et. al. 2000/2002).

Along with TBW, endurance trained athletes generally posess a higher BV (besides smaller fat and body mass) compared to untrained subjects (Grund et. al. 2001). The enlargement of BV already exerts after a few days of prolonged exercise and takes several months to develop (Fellmann 1992, Fellmann et. al. 1999, Guglielmini et. al. 1989, Schmidt et. al. 1988/1989/2000, Schumacher et. al. 2000/2002). During the first two weeks of training nearly all BV gain can be explained by PV expansion while there is no change in red blood cell mass. After this initial period a continuous increase in erythrocyte volume occurs, leading to a rebalancing of Hb and Hct concentrations to pre training level due to the new, more equally distributed plasma and erythrocyte volume (Convertino 1980/1983/1991, Sawka et. al. 2000, Schmidt et. al. 1989).

Due to the more pronounced PV expansion, levels of Hb and Hct fall as a long term consequence of aerobic endurance training as well as repeated bouts of strenuous exercise, e. g. repetitive cycling races or cycling stage races over several consecutive days during the competitive season (ADA 2009a, Convertino 1983/1991, Fellmann 1992, Kleiner 1999, Leiper et. a. 2001, Neumayr et. al. 2002a/2003b, Saris et. al. 1998, Schumacher et. al. 2000/2002, Wirnitzer and Faulhaber 2007). However, Convertino (1991), Fellmann et. al. (1999) and Sawka et. al. (2000) found that PV expansion peaked on the fourth day of multiple day endurance races.

An increase in BV normally results in enhanced aerobic performance due to reduced blood viscosity, thereby optimized microcirculation and improved oxygen delivery capacity to the working muscle (Schumacher et. al. 2000). However, the exercise induced effect of HR decline may be closely related to cardiovascular changes and PV expansion. The latter allows a better venous return that generates a rise of end diastolic volume and an enhancement of stroke volume. Consequently, the same cardic output as before could be maintained with a lower HR (Convertino 1980/1983/1991, Mounier et. al. 2003, Sawka et. al. 2000). Both Convertino (1983) and Mounier et. al. (2003) found PV increase and HR reduction to be closely related (+1 % in PV is linked to −1 % in HR), pointing out a significant relationship between the individual changes in PV and HR in cycling.

The current results strengthen the role of PV expansion in HR decline, showing the drop in mean HR to be linked to extended PV (Stage 4: –5.4 % in HR along with +5.5 % in PV; Stage 6: –6.7 % in HR along with +6.9 % in PV), respectively compared to Stage 1.

During endurance exercise both the volume and distribution of body fluids are challenged by thermoregulatory, hydrostatic and osmotic perturbations. When exposed to heat stress (metabolic and/or thermal) during prolonged strenuous exercise, an additional rise in metabolism and body temperature is generated (Convertino 1980/1983, Sawka et. al. 2000, Schumacher et. al. 2000/2002; for more detail see Chapter 4.3. Nutritional strategies – Vegan nutrition pattern). Thus, heat elimination causes a peripheral redistribution of blood flow (Savard et. al. 1988) and leads to body fluid shifts between water pools (Harrison 1985). As a result of thermoregulation, athletes may lose a considerable amount of body water due to elevated sweat rate and respiration. The subsequent PV decline leads to enhanced levels of Hb and Hct (Convertino 1991, Mounier et. al. 2003, Sawka et. al. 2000, Schmidt et. al. 2000, Schumacher et. al. 2000). Body water decrements of as little as 1 – 3 % of body mass have adverse effects on exercise performance (ADA 2009a, De Marees 2003, Leiper et. al. 2001).

Together, these factors result in reduced BV during cycling exercise in heat and, thereby, reduce the available blood to perfuse the working muscles (Maw et. al. 1996). Hypohydration status has usually been obtained after heat exposure, exercise or a combination of both (Koulmann et. al. 2000, O`Brien et. al. 2002). Koulmann et. al. (2000) studied acute changes in body fluid compartments (TBW, ECW) after heat and exercise induced dehydration. The decline in TBW is greatest for heat, while the fall in ECW is twofold higher in heat compared to exercise. Heat induced and exercise induced dehydration show a decrease in ECW nearly representing the same decline in TBW (heat: 37 % versus exercise: 36 %). Generally, hemoconcentration is documented to be accompanied by enhanced blood viscosity. To compensate the lower circulating BV, HR must increase in order to maintain a constant cardic output and, consequenty, an adequate oxygen supply for muscle demand (Galy et. al. 2005, Schumacher et. al., 2000/2002).

Adequate fluid substitution is crucial to maintain optimal physiological and psychological performance (Kleiner 1999, Martinoli et. al. 2003, Sawka et. al. 2007, Shanholtzer and Patterson 2003; for more detail see Chapter 4.4. Mood and mental capacity) and to successfully participate in marathon races. Athletes should replace large amounts of fluid by constantly repeated FI (nibbling character) during daily stages in order to avoid dehydration (Jeukendrup 2002a, Hargreaves et. al. 1996a).

Acute variations in haematological levels are based on changes in PV due to fluid filtrations following osmotic gradients and/or increased hydrostatic pressure (Convertino 1980/1983/1991, Galy et. al. 2005, Guglielmini et. al. 1989, Mounier et. al. 2003, Sawka et. al. 2000, Schmidt et. al. 2000, Schumacher et. al. 2000/2002). These temporary responses, caused by body water losses, are nearly gone after recovery period. A faster rebound to pre exercise fluid volumes and haematological levels could be explained by the better capacity of recovery in well endurance trained athletes compared to normal subjects (Neumayr et. al. 2005).

Following these findings it can be suggested that acute shifts in body water and haematological status probably occurred due to combination of both exercise and heat induced dehydration during Stage 1, but was balanced by adequate hydration strategy during recovery period between consecutive stages of TAC 2004.

While acute exercise on a short term basis generally leads to hemoconcentration, long term exercise may causes hemodilution (Neumayr et. al. 2002a). Due to the long time preparation focusing the TAC as the main event of the MTB season, it can be supposed that PV expansion has already been occurred even before this severe stage race as a result of endurance training over a period of several months to almost a year. Moreover, ultraendurance events are known to induce a transient hypervolemia during the recovery period, which already occurs some hours after a single bout of exercise and usually returns to its initial level within five to seven days (Convertino 1991, Fellmann 1992, Fellmann et. al. 1999, Schmidt et. al. 1988/1989/2000). Furthermore, body composition changes could be counterbalanced mainly due to a loss of fat mass, resulting in a constant body mass and even, in some cases, in a body mass increase (Pialoux et. al. 2004, Pivarnik et. al. 1984).

Thus, it might be suggested that MTB athletes, who had an extended PV in the morning before the initial start of the TAC 2004 as well as each subsequent stage (secondary hypervolemia), could benefit from theses adaptations during daily competition. These data, although representing a small number of athletes, are evident that due to exercise induced chronic PV expansion, well endurance trained competitive MTBers might be rather characterized by lower Hb and Hct values than an untrained comparative population (Saris et. al. 1998, Schmidt et. al. 2000)

4.1.4. Prerequisites for the Transalp Challenge

Knowledge of the physiological requirements necessary to successfully participate in MTB events is crucial to develop adequate training strategies and tactics during MTB stage racing.

The current findings demonstrate that a TAC puts a severe impact on the cardiovascular system due to a daily UCI XCM race over eight successive stages. Thus, the training has to be individually planned and carried out both high in extent and intensity. The afore mentioned completely unique profile of skills, physiological characteristics and race induced impact distribution needs to be met by MTB–specific training to cope with all the requirements that an off–road cyclist has to face. Since the TAC is the premier MTB event of the XCM race calendar, some athletes might participate in the TAC only once in their life. Competing in severe MTB stage races might be possible after a minimal training for 4 – 6 weeks, but is not advisable. Therefore, participation at the start of the TAC has to be well prepared for and takes time to reach an adequate level of performance to meet this challenge.

The prerequisites to compete in and probably finish a TAC are a high level in both anaerobic and aerobic power and capacity.

Anaerobic power and capacity. MTBing requires both endurance and sprint abilities. Therefore, success in MTB racing is suggested to depend to a large proportion on anaerobic power and capacity (Faria et. al. 2005a, Impellizzeri and Marcora 2007). In order to determine anaerobic ability the athlete is required to generate as much work as possible (seated position, 50 – 140 rpm) during 10 – 30 seconds of isokinetic cycle sprinting (Faria et. al. 2005a). The test most frequently used is the Wingate standard protocol (30–second sprint test; Faria et. al. 2005b, Palmer 2002). PPO and average PO in this 30 second sprint test equate to anaerobic power (the peak PO generated) and anaerobic capacity (the total PO that the muscle can produce using anaerobic sources) (Faria et. al. 2005b, Palmer 2002). The cyclists ability to generate high PO of brief duration is of great importance at the start of a race (Stapelfeldt et. al. 2004), during the uphill climbs, while passing counterparts or slower riders, and finally while sprinting to the finish (Faria et. al. 2005a). Therefore, high PPO (absolute and relative to body mass) is an essential prerequisite to MTB success (Faria et. al. 2005b). PPO of MTBers have been found to be 14.9 W/kg (national and international level: Baron 2001) and of 14.2 W/kg (national level, unpublished data: Impellizzeri and Marcora 2007).

Aerobic power and capacity. MTB races are suggested to require high rates of aerobic energy production (Impellizzeri et. al. 2002, Stapelfeldt et. al. 2004, Wirnitzer and Kornexl 2008, Wirnitzer 2009a+b). Basically, cycling puts extremely high aerobic demands on the athletes both at maximal and submaximal exercise intensities. A cyclists performance potential is determined by the evaluation of absolute performance related measures, including maximum aerobic power (PO_{MAX}), maximum oxygen uptake (VO_{2MAX}) and blood lactate levels. However, the aerobic performance level can be more accurately predicted when physiological measures are expressed as relative values (Mujika and Padilla 2002, Palmer 2002).

It is generally suggested that a high PO_{MAX} and VO_{2MAX} might be beneficial to endurance performance (Coyle et. al. 1991, Mujika and Padilla 2002, Palmer 2002).

Several studies demonstrate that MTBers can utilise a high percentage of their PO_{MAX} to produce the high and prolonged work rates required (Impellizzeri et. al. 2002/2005a, Lee et. al. 2002, MacRae et. al. 2000, Wilber et. al. 1997). PO at LT2 has been shown to be an important variable in cycling performance (Coyle et. al. 1991, Faria 2005a). LT4 (identified as the exercise intensity eliciting a blood lactate concentration of 4 mmol/L: Faria 2005a) has been reported as the highest possible steady state work intensity that can be maintained for a prolonged period of time. Therefore, PO at LT4 is an excellent indicator of a cyclist`s endurance potential (Faria 2005a).

Maximum oxygen uptake is considered to be a valid indicator of the integrated function of respiratory, cardiovascular and muscular systems during exercise and an important determinant of endurance performance (Impellizzeri and Marcora 2007).

High level MTBers have been shown to possess a high VO_{2MAX} ranging from 76.9 – 78.3 mL/kg*min (Impellizzeri et. al. 2005b, Lee et. al. 2002) while mean values of 66.5 – 75.9 mL/kg*min were found in elite MTBers (Baron 2001, Impellizzeri et. al. 2002/2005a, Nishii et. al. 2004, Stapelfeldt et. al. 2004, Warner et. al. 2002, Wilber et. al. 1997). In amateur MTBers, values of VO_{2MAX} ranging from 56.6 – 60.0 mL/kg*min (Berry et. al. 2000, Cramp et. al. 2004, MacRae et. al. 2000) have been reported.

The intensity profile of MTBers suggest that an athlete should be able to sustain high work rates for a prolonged period of time. This has been confirmed by several studies on the ventilatory and lactate threshold. The LT (defined as exponential increase in blood lactate concentration above baseline in response to progressive submaximal workloads) has been shown to correspond to 75 – 77 % of VO_{2MAX} in national team members and elite MTBers (Impellizzeri et. al. 2002/2005a, MacRae et. al. 2000, Wilber et. al. 1997). In top level Australian MTBers Lee et. al. (2002) measured an LT (modified D–max method) corresponding to 86 % of VO_{2MAX}. Moreover, Impellizzeri et. al. (2002/2005a) reported intensities at onset of blood lactate accumulation (LT4) corresponding to 85 – 89 % of VO_{2MAX}.

Taken together, this results in submaximal economy which is most easily defined as the oxygen cost to work at a given intensity. The ability of a well trained athlete to sustain a high economy of motion, is described as the least amount of oxygen possible used to produce the highest work by the muscle (Palmer 2002). The higher the efficiency, the lower the oxygen cost to work at a given intensity will be. Simultaneously, an increase in endurance level occurs (Mujika and Padilla 2002, Palmer 2002).

Figure 22. Uphill climb during Stage 4 (Bressanone/ITA to St. Christina/ITA) of the Transalp Challenge 2009 (© JEANTEX BIKE TRANSALP powered by NISSAN – Peter Musch, with permission from 3rd August 2009).

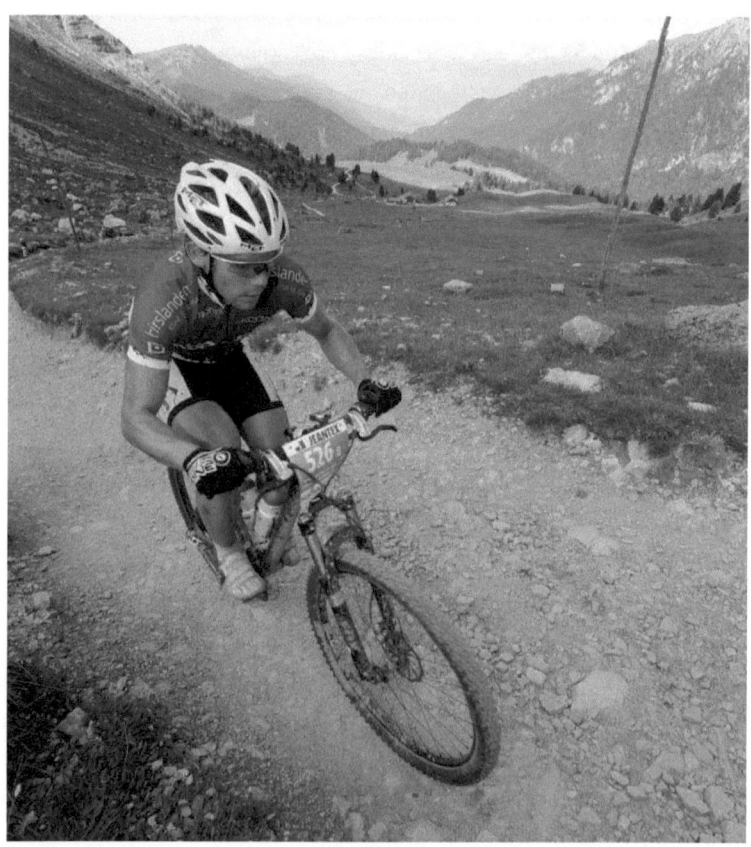

4.2. Bike handling mastery and race tactics

Additionally, experienced bike handling is essential to the final ranking in MTB sports. During downhill sections a MTB athlete can defend or extend the runtime gap to other competitors.

The Olympic XC and XCM as well as the TAC are characterised by a great diversity of terrains and traits, where single tracks are technically very difficult. Therefore, during off–road cycling intense and repeated isometric contractions of arm and leg muscles are necessary to absorb shock and vibrations and for bike handling and stabilization. This might lead to a permanently elevated HR, especially in downhill sections performed on rough terrains (Hurst and Atkins 2002/2006, Impellizzeri et. al. 2002, Seifert et. al. 1997, Stapelfeldt et. al. 2004, Wang and Hull 1997).

Similarly to uphill climbing (88 % HR_{MAX}Field), the downhill sections are also physiologically and mentally very demanding (78 % HR_{MAX}Field). For that reason, in sections performed on rough terrains, especially in technical elements during downhill, elevated HR might be explained due to a high level of concentration and the additional mental stress (Hurst and Atkins 2002/2006, Impellizzeri et. al. 2002/2005a+b/2008, Stapelfeldt et. al. 2004, Wang and Hull 1997). These requirements are necessarily needed to be met by a competent bike handling. Professional MTBers, such as the professional MTB athlete and 7 times winner of TAC Karl Platt (Germany), still improve their high level of bike handling mastery under the guidance of professional instructors.

Usually, the circuit of XC races is reasonably well known by covering a specific number of identical loops on the same course. Thus, the athlete is familiar with the technical difficulties of the XC course. By contrast, the course of the TAC is always new and unknown. Therefore, the effect of habituation that might be advantageous in XC competitions, can be excluded for competing in the TAC.

HR have been shown to be close to maximum values immediately after the start as the initial phase in MTB races is crucial for overall performance and final ranking. MTBers try to place themselves in the front positions to avoid slowing down when the path narrows into single track trails and overtaking becomes difficult (Impellizzeri et. al. 2002, Impellizzeri and Marcora 2007, Stapelfeldt et. al. 2004). Moreover, some riders increase their speed downhill where MTBers can gain advantage or decrease time lost in other parts of the course. It is suggested that small differences in technical ability and bike handling mastery between riders could be crucial for performance among physiologically similar MTBers (Impellizzeri and Marcora 2007).

In road cycling, race tactics are mainly determined by the team tactics of supporting the team leader or specialist (e. g. uphill climb, team time trial). Briefly, drafting reduces energy cost of road cycling by as much as 40 %. Likewise there is a 40 % reduction of air resistance when drafting in the middle of the pack. This reduced drag force has the effect of lowering the oxygen uptake, HR, ventilation and lactate values while cycling in comparison to remaining at the front (Faria et. al. 2005b). In contrast to road cycling, in MTB sports the exercise intensity is not affected by bunch building and/or drafting, but is determined by each athletes' individual performance.

Figure 23. Bike handling mastery, during uphill climb, but especially during downhill sections (with permission from 27th July 2009), is essential to overall ranking in MTB races.

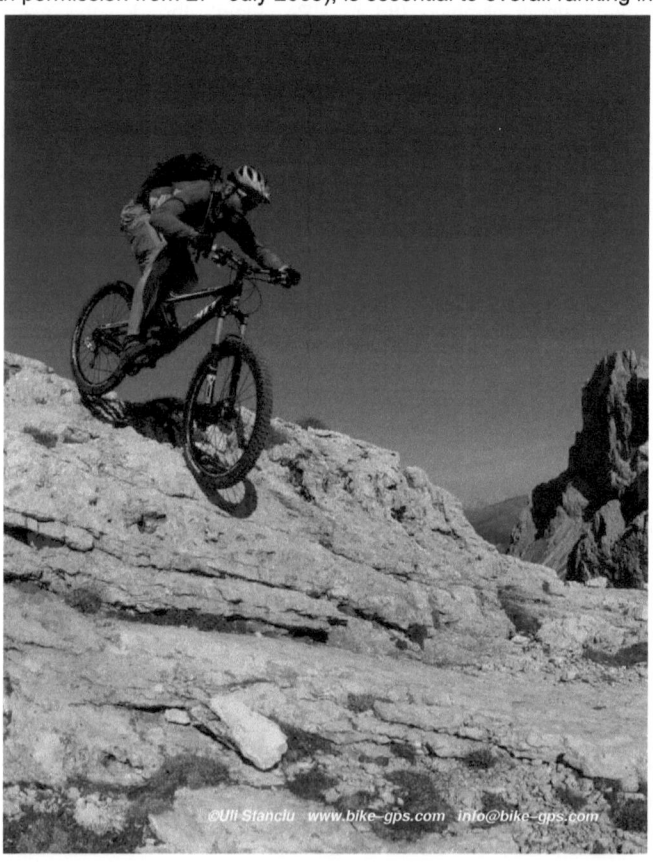

4.3. Nutritional strategies – Vegan nutrition pattern

Nutritional treatment is well known to play a major role in endurance performance. Optimum performance cannot be maintained without adequate glycogen stores based on appropriate diet, especially during competition.

"It is the position of the American Dietetic Association, Dietitians of Canada, and the American College of Sports Medicine that physical activity, athletic performance, and recovery from exercise are enhanced by optimal nutrition. These organizations recommend appropriate selection of food and fluids, timing of intake, and supplement of choices for optimal health and exercise performance" (ADA 2009a).

To complete the TAC, tremendous strains have to be accomplished and vast amounts of energy have to be replaced. Therefore, careful planning and monitoring of nutrient intake is required to meet the energy demands of MTB stage racing. To the best of the author's knowledge, no studies have yet examined the dietary intake during MTB XCM or stage racing.

Since vegetarian and vegan nutrition strategies were introduced to high performance sports and women have begun competing in the same MTB races as men, information about the requirements of the vegetarian and vegan cyclist as well as recommendations for the dietary intake of female road and off–road cyclists have become important. The use of current dietary recommendations for female athletes is limited as they have been developed from male athletic populations (Gabel 2002). In general, data on female cyclists is sparse and insufficient, if available at all (Burke 2001).

Protein – a historical review. In 1839 the Dutch chemist Gerhard Mulder discovered the nitrogen–containing chemical substance protein (Greek: proteios, "of premium importance"; Campbell and Campbell 2006). Justus von Liebig, the preeminent physiological chemist at that time, promoted the concept of protein oxidation to produce the energy for all muscular movement (Liebig 1842, Nieman 1988). Soon, the subsequent research (1850s and 1860s) has shown this theory as to be false by detecting CHO and fat as the major fuel of muscular activity (Nieman 1988). Despite this, early scientists such as the German Carl Voit were staunch advocates of protein. He stated that "man" cannot get too much protein. Voit was the mentor of several nutritional scientists in the early 1900s, such as Wilbur O. Atwater (organizer and director of the first nutrition laboratory at the United States Department of Agriculture, USA). The British physician Major McCay was stationed in the colony of India (1912). By identifying good fighting men in the Indian tribes, he commented that people who consumed less protein were found to be of worse physique (Campbell and Campbell 2006).

To date, protein is still the most misunderstood and misinterpreted of all nutrients. In the 19th century protein was synonymous with animal protein. Protein was, and today still is, equated with meat. The vital force was suggested to be exclusively inserted into meat. Therefore, the people were encouraged to eat as much meat as possible. The belief in this connection is still held by many people. Most people immediately think of meat, when they consider protein. That is why vegetarians and vegans still have to face the question of how they will obtain their protein requirements, because plant based protein is even thought to be execrable (Campbell and Campbell 2006).

Following the accumulated scientific knowledge of the past, someone ate plenty of protein (meat), if he/she was civilized and rich. When a person was poor and belonged to the lower social classes, they ate plant based foods such as potatoes and bread. They were considered to be indolent and less capable, as a result of not eating sufficient amounts of animal protein. As a consequence, this misguided awareness of the past centuries leaded to a fundamental cultural bias that had become firmly entrenched (Campbell and Campbell 2006).

Scientific studies considering plant based nutrition connected to sports. The relationship between nutrition and exercise has been a major area of scientific interest for over 150 years (Febbraio 2002).

In the mid–to–late 1800s, vegetarians sought to prove through excellence in endurance exercise the superiority of a plant based diet. During the 1890s, the London Vegetarian Society formed an athletic and cycling club to compete against their meat eating counterparts. Vegetarian athletes outperformed the latter in most cases during competition. In 1896, the Vegetarian Cycling Club (90 members including 13 women) gained easy victory over two regular clubs. Amongst these, a vegetarian cyclist won the most prestigious hill–climbing race in England by breakding the hill record by nearly a minute. Also an American vegetarian cyclist broke all records for the 3219–km bicycle race and a vegetarian female established a women's record for 1609 km (Nieman 1988, Whorton 1982).

At the beginning of the 20th century, approximately at the same time, some few researchers (Chittenden 1904/1907, Fisher 1907, Ioteyko 1906/1907/1911 and Schouteden 1904) studied how vegetarian diets are related to exercise performance.

Russell H. Chittenden, a well established scientist in the field of nutrition at the Yale University Medical School, studied whether the consumption of plant based diets influences physical capacities. The physical performance of the male subjects (students, fellow faculty members, himself) was measured during laboratory testing. He found that ingesting a plant based diet enables the subject to exercise more, with less fatigue, compared with a diet based on animal protein (Chittenden 1904/1907). Simultaneously at Yale, Irving Fisher (having a wide range of interests including diet and nutrition) designed a series of tests to compare the stamina and strength of meat–eaters against those of vegetarians. Male subjects were selected from three groups: meat–eating athletes, vegetarian athletes and vegetarian sedentary subjects. In the horizontal arm–hold test for example, 22 of 32 vegetarians exceeded 15 minutes, 15 broke 30 minutes, 9 broke 60 minutes and 1 subject surpassed 3 hours. Conversely, only 2 of 15 meat eaters were able to maintain a duration of more than 15 minutes while none reached the 30 minutes mark. The accumulated results have shown that vegetarians have twice the stamina of meat eaters, showing the latter to have far less endurance than the vegetarians (even in sedentary subjects). He reasoned that the difference in endurance was entirely due to the difference in their diet. He provided strong evidence that a vegetarian diet raises endurance (Fisher 1907).

The Belgian researcher H. Schouteden conducted tests in 25 male subjects, divided into two groups of vegetarians and meat–eaters. The number of times that vegetarians and meat–eaters could lift a weight by squeezing a handle (right hand) was compared. The mean number of contractions achieved by the vegetarians was 69, while the meat–eaters averaged 38. As in all former studies which have measured time to muscle recovery, the vegetarians bounced back from fatigue far more rapidly than did the meat eaters did (Schouteden 1904, Berry 1909).

Josefa Ioteyko (Academie de Medicine de Paris) compared the endurance of vegetarians and meat–eaters from all walks of life in a variety of tests. The vegetarians (43 subjects) averaged two to three times more endurance than that shown by the meat eaters. Even more remarkably, they took one fifth of the time to recover from exhaustion than the meat eating group did (Ioteyko and Kipiani 1906/1907, Ioteyko 1911).

In 1968, a Danish team of researchers re–popularized Fishers classic Yale study. A variety of diets were tested on male subjects by using a stationary bicycle to measure their strength and endurance. First, the men were fed a mixed diet of meat and vegetables for a period of time, and then tested on the bicycle. The average time they could pedal before muscle failure was 114 minutes. Later, they were fed a diet rich in meat, milk and eggs for a similar period and were then re-tested. On the high animal protein diet, their pedalling time dropped dramatically to 57 minutes. Finally, the group was switched to a strictly vegetarian diet, composed of grains, vegetables and fruits. Following a diet lacking in animal products, they pedalled for an average of 167 minutes (Astrand 1968).

Growing interest in vegetarian diets. Hardinge and Crooks (1963) have been the first who (representatively, rather than exhaustedly) reviewed the scientific literature related to vegetarian nutrition by evaluating the early literature up to 1962 (96 reports predominantly in English language). Since the late 1960s, there has been a sharp growth in professional interest in vegetarian nutrition (Figure 24). The number of articles in the scientific literature related to vegetarism (average of 8 in 1966 to 76 in 1995) has increased steadily, almost linearily, during 30 years (Sabate et. al. 1999). Additionally, the main focus of the articles is changing. In the late 1960s, articles primarily tended to question the nutritional adequacy of vegetarian diets. More recently, the predominant issue has been the use of vegetarian diets in the prevention and treatment of chronic disease. There is a growing appreciation of the clear benefits of plant-based diets (ADA 2003/2009a+b, Campbell and Campbell 2006).

In 1978, the earliest major report on five studies which measured the diets of a cohort of individuals and monitored their subsequent death was published. It compared disease mortality in pure vegetarians (vegans) with that in other vegetarians and meat-eaters. The results showed the vegans to have had the lowest rates of mortality due to heart disease. Along with other studies, this confirmed the vegetarian diets to be beneficial against heart disease (Phillips et. al. 1978).

Figure 24. Development of scientific interest in vegetarian nutrition, contrasting the early years up to 1962 (pooled and drawn after Hardinge and Crooks 1963, Berry 1909, Chittenden 1907, Ioteyko and Kipiani 1906/1907, Ioteyko 1911, Schouteden 1904) to the number of articles published per year more recently (1966 – 1995: Sabate et. al. 1999).

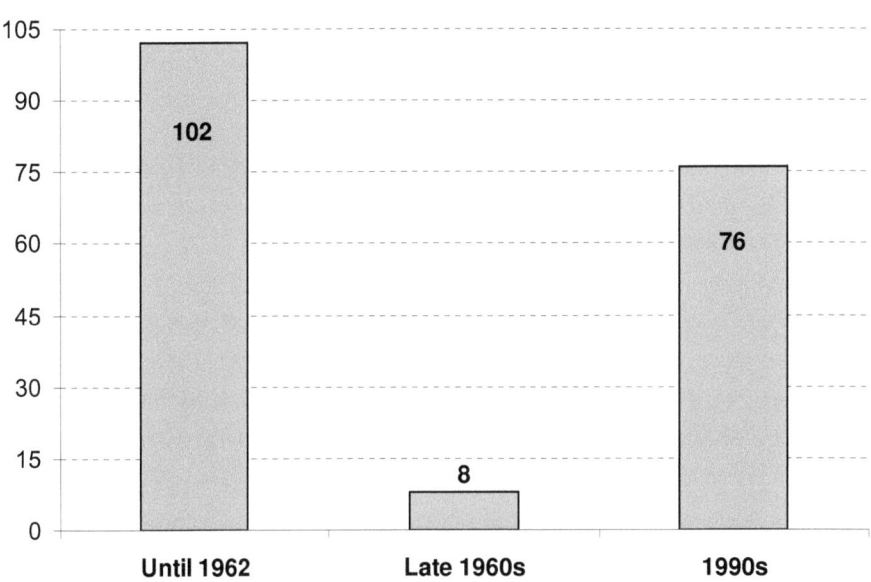

Racing in the heat. When exercising in the heat, in addition to endogenous heat being produced, thermoregulatory mechanisms of the body are heavily stressed by heat loss. As a result fatigue prior to CHO depletion occurs. Therefore, fluid ingestion is of major importance in order to postpone a rise in body core temperature and to prevent impaired exercise performance resulting from several factors (Febbraio 2002). Any athlete who is exposed to heat may require different levels of some nutrients from those recommended by current guidelines (Knechtle et. al. 2005). It is generally accepted that exercise in the heat results in a substrate shift towards increased CHO utilization (Febbraio 2002).

FI not only attenuates the rise in body core temperature, it also reduces the likelihood of CHO depletion by reducing the muscle glycogen use during prolonged exercise (Hargreaves et. al. 1996a+b). Together, both CHO and fluid availability are vital when exposed to heat during severe exercise and result in an improved exercise performance in a hot environment (Below et. al. 1995, Febbraio 2002). Therefore, especially during racing, it is important to maintain appropriate FI and adequate energy supply to fuel muscle contraction and to prevent both hyperthermia and exercise induced dehydration.

The levels of exercise induced FI, as well as the markedly high values of CHO intake during daily racing and whole TAC 2004, seem to be appropriate to sustain the high effort of this stage race, considering the hot and dry conditions faced by the subject together with the high exercise intensity.

Off–road cycling. Ultraendurance cycling and stage racing poses an increased demand for energy and CHO. Meeting these demands requires careful planning and monitoring of dietary intake (Lindemann 1991).

In addition to heat exposure, the high EI found during the TAC 2004 can be explained by the characteristics of XC competitions as previously discussed. Particularly during MTB races, FI and EI are usually limited by the practical situation. The nutritional requirements of a TAC are challenging for several reasons. Opportunities and time available for FI and EI are restricted by a great diversity of terrains and traits (difficult nature of course profile during both uphill and downhill sections) simultaneously with aggressive riding tactics (Wirnitzer and Kornexl 2008, Wirnitzer 2009a+b). In contrast to road cycling, downhill sections are not sections of either low intensity or recovery (Hurst and Atkins 2002/2006, Stapelfeldt et. al. 2004) and therefore dietary intake is almost impossible. Despite these factors combining to prevent the athlete from consuming more food and drinks, the nutritional requirements necessarily had to be met by appropriate dietary intake. As a consequence, a greater reliance was put on post race replenishment to provide EI, mainly through CHO as the most important fuel in ultraendurance and cycling (stage) races.

Information on the effects of dietary interventions on MTB performance is scarce. Recently, Rose and Peters (2008) studied amateur MTBers during a three days MTB race (Sani2C MTB Race, South Africa) in cool conditions (6 – 21 °C). Wingo et. al. (2004) examined the influence of pre–exercise glycerol drinks on performance and physiologic function in a one day XC MTB race in the heat. Cramp et. al. (2004) conducted a simulated MTB race in the laboratory (93 min) to study the effects of consuming different CHO treatments on metabolic effects and performance. Mastroianni et. al. (2000) studied the differences in energy expenditure between off–road cyclists and runners while voluntarily pacing. Seifert el. al. (1997) investigated the energy cost of riding a full versus front suspended MTB. In these studies all the subjects were male. Due to the wide range of purposes, conditions and design of these few studies available, the current findings are difficult to use for comparative purposes.

Major stage races and ultraendurance cycling. Several authors have described the dietary practice of athletes during major cycling tours. The few studies available report mean daily EIs of 23.3 MJ (Erp van–Baart et. al. 1989: Tour l'Avenir), 23.5 MJ (Garcia–Roves et. al. 1998) and 24.7 MJ (Saris et. al. 1989) for male athletes competing in the major stage races. Maximum values of EI were found of 28.2 MJ/day were found during the Vuelta a Espana (Garcia–Roves et. al. 1998) and of 32.4 MJ/day during the Tour de France (Saris et. al. 1989). The relative contributions of energy from CHO, protein and fat was similar during both the Tour de France (Saris et. al. 1989: 62 %, 15 % and 23 %) and the Vuelta a Espana (Garcia–Roves et. al. 1998: 60 %, 14.5 % and 25.5 %). In contrast to the TAC 2004, cyclists in the Tour de France consumed 49 % of their total EI during the race. Moreover, 58 % of daily CHO ingested was taken during daily stages. About 30 % of total CHO intake came from CHO rich liquids. Mean daily FI was 6.7 L with 61 % (4.1 L) of total fluid consumed during daily racing in the Tour de France (Saris et. al. 1989).

During the Race Across America (RAAM) the relative contribution of total calories consumed from CHO as the main source of energy was found to be 75.2 % (Knechtle et. al. 2005) and 78 % (Lindemann 1991). Since environmental conditions were similar for the RAAM (Lindemann 1991: 21 – 35 °C) and TAC 2004, mean FI resulted in 0.72 L/h runtime and 0.57 L/h runtime, respectively.

The relative contribution of CHO to total EI in the TAC 2004 exceeds the results of the Tour de France and Vuelta a Espana, but was quite comparable to those of RAAM.

Dietary intake during TAC 2004. In the course of the TAC 2004 the subject gradually become weary of the sweet taste of energy food and drinks ingested during the race. Therefore, spicy food and dishes were preferred, especially post race. Even though the cyclist permanently felt sated, she tried to eat constantly to provide energy replenishment and to restore muscle glycogen. Since the energy cost of cycling is an exponential function of speed (Jeukendrup 2002b) the average speed during TAC 2004 (15.6 km/h) is connected to the high EI of 24.6 MJ/day. The body mass measured after daily stages remained stable after oscillating from stages 1 to 4. This indicates that CHO replacement and hydration strategies were adequate.

Pre race. Except for Stage 1, which had a unique start time of 12 a. m., breakfast was daily taken at 6.30 a. m. due to the early start times of 8 a. m. It is suprising that only once gastrointenstinal discomfort did occur, during breakfast of Stage 7, resulting in the lowest EI. Compared to the major stage races of road cycling, where start times are fixed at around noon, the time for dietary intake prior to the race was very limited. As a consequence, pre race values for EI and FI were found to be low in the TAC 2004. Fluid consumed was approximately half the volume of 300 – 400 mL recommended to be consumed pre race (Jeukendrup 2002a). CHO intake during breakfast fitted well with the pre race recommendations of Burke (2002: 1 – 4 g CHO/kg) with 49 – 196 g CHO derived for the subject.

Race. The fluid ingested during the race, exclusively coming from sport drinks rich in CHO, fits well with the current recommendations for both CHO solution (Maughan 2002: 2 – 8 %) and relative FI during races lasting more than 90 min (Jeukendrup 2002a: 8 – 12 mL/kg*h), with volumes of 400 – 600 mL/h ingested for the MTBer. On the one hand, the findings for CHO intake during daily racing (479 g) exceed the recommendations of 60 – 70 g CHO/h runtime (Burke 2002, Hargreaves 2002, Jeukendrup 2002a) with derived values of 315 – 368 g CHO. On the other hand, total daily CHO intake during stage races lasting more than 4 – 5 hours of high intensity cycling is 12 – 13 g/kg reported for male cyclists (Burke 2001). The fact that the subject was a non–professional female is likely to explain the considerably lower amount of CHO consumed.

Post race. Following the experience gained by competing the TAC in 2003, sleeping time was strictly held from 10 p. m. to 6 a. m. in order to maximize recovery. Quick recovery is extremely important during stage races. The replenishment of muscle glycogen stores and fluid balance to pre race levels after daily competition is probably the most important factor (Jeukendrup 2002a). To maximize glycogen storage, the ingestion of CHO rich fluids and easily digestible solid CHO rich foods such as bananas, is preferred (Brouns et. al. 1986, Jentjens 2002, Jeukendrup 2002a). Even when CHO intake between successive days of racing is very high, the muscle glycogen levels might be suboptimal when the CHO need is critically high and when the next stage is started within 8 – 16 hours (Jentjens 2002, Jeukendrup 2002a). Since the female in the TAC 2004 was usually riding for 4 – 7 hours daily, there was barely enough time for eating large meals. However, the challenges posed be the practical constraints, both in terms of the limited time available for eating and the suppression of appetite after exhaustive exercise (Brouns et. al. 1986, Burke 2001, Jeukendrup 2002a+b), appear to have been met by the subject. Relative daily post race ingestion from CHO nicely meets the recommendations for stage races with 5 – 6 h of extreme endurance effort of 1 – 1.2 g CHO/kg*h (Jentjens 2002, Jeukendrup 2002a). Derived ranges for the MTB athlete (490 – 590 g CHO/day) fits well with current results (529 g CHO). Contrary to road cycling, the most important occasions to eat were post exercise.

Energy intake from macronutrients. Compared to guidelines for endurance trained female athletes, fat intake (9.2 % of total EI) was found to be about half the recommended intake (ADA 2009a, Gabel 2002: 20 – 35 % of total EI) and relative protein intake was about twice the recommended levels (ADA 2009a, Lemon 1995: 1.2 – 1.4 g protein/kg*day). Protein requirements of endurance athletes are known to exceed those of recreational subjects (Gabel 2002). The mean daily intakes of protein and micronutrients are likely to meet or exceed advocated levels for the MTBer competing in TAC 2004, largely because of high EIs (Burke 2001, Saris et. al. 1989).

Martin et. al. (2002) studied the EI (self reported) and energy expenditure in eight elite female cyclists (members of the Australian national training squad: 25 years, 59 kg) during eight days of training and racing, including a five days stage race. They reported a mean EI of 14.87 MJ/day. During five days of racing, intake from fat and protein was reported to have been 59 g/day and 136 g/day, respectively. These values correspond with the current findings of fat (58 g/day) and protein (107 g/day).

Carbohydrate. The importance of CHO as a main source of fuel for performance during prolonged endurance exercise has been recognized since the 1930s (Jentjens 2002). Christensen and Hansen (1939a+b) were among the first to demonstrate the influence of CHO on improving or maintaining exercise performance during exercise. CHO replacement plays an essential role during prolonged intensive cycling races (Burke 2001). The oxidation of CHO can provide energy at a faster rate than fat oxidation. Therefore, CHO is the preferred fuel at exercise intensities higher than 80 % of maximum HR when large amounts of energy have to be generated over long periods of time (Burke 2001, Jeukendrup 2002b). Suitable food choices to attain such goals include concentrated sport drinks and portable CHO rich foods such as solid energy bars and gels (Brouns et. al. 1986, Jeukendrup 2002a). CHO ingestion during exercise has been shown to improve race performance in events of more than 90 min of duration by maintaining both high levels of both plasma glucose and CHO oxidation. The increased availability of plasma glucose enables the athlete to postpone fatigue or to develop a higher PO in a final sprint following endurance exercise (Coggan and Coyle 1987/1988/1989, Hargreaves et. al. 1984). A further mechanism to improve cycling performance by CHO ingestion might be also the resynthesis of muscle glycogen during periods of low intensity (Hargreaves et. al. 1984, Jeukendrup 2002a).

In the current study, an intake of 1195 g/day came from CHO. Compared to Martin et. al. (2002), who reported a CHO intake of 588 g/day during a race period of five days, the result of the MTBer is about twice the value of that for female road cyclists. Erp van–Baart et. al. (1989), studying amateur cyclists in the Tour l`Avenir reported a daily intake of 873 g from CHO. Almost a decade later, Garcia–Roves et. al. (1998) found a similar CHO intake during the Vuelta a Espana (841.4 g/day). Currently recommended energy from CHO for a more competitive woman participating in endurance and ultra endurance events had been given as 55 – 70 % of total intake (Gabel 2002). The total calories coming from CHO during TAC 2004 (83.3 %) exceed the advocated range by about 13.3 %. Relative CHO intake (24.4 g/kg*day) is twice as high as the recommendations of 8 – 12 g CHO/kg*day (Jentjens 2002, Jeukendrup 2002a) and more than twice the guidelines for female athletes of 6 – 10 g CHO/kg per day (Gabel 2002).

Dietary intake in vegan athletes. The vegan diet is determined to be exclusively sourced from plant based nutrition, rejecting all products from animal sources (as one unit, ingredient or supplement) such as meat, fish, dairy products, egg and honey (Figure 25).

Figure 25. Vegan nutrition pyramide after Petter and Pohlmann (2007; with permission from 2nd December 2008).

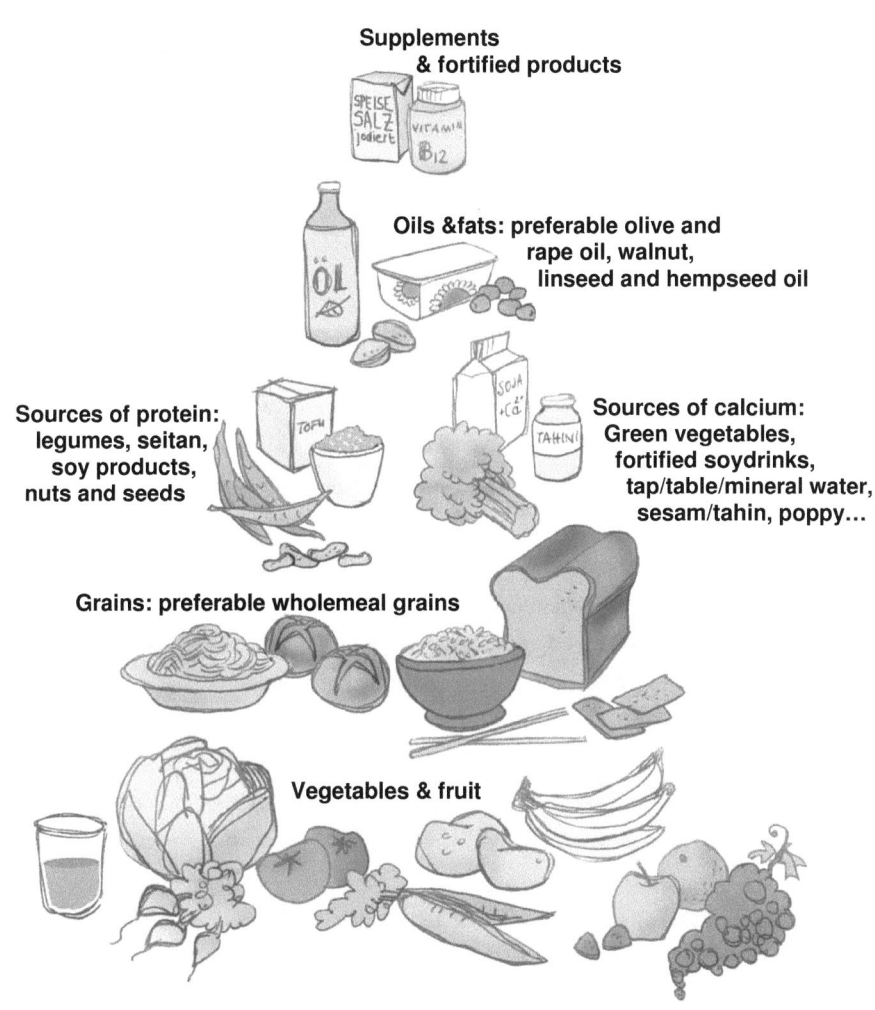

The European Union currently has 1.73 % of its population (6.72 million people) following a vegetarian or vegan lifestyle (representative survey conducted by the European Commission: http://ec.europa.eu/food/animal/welfare/euro_barometer25_volA_en.pdf). A UK wide survey carried out by the Food Standards Agency (Consumer Attitudes to Food Standards 2007: www.vegsoc.org/info/statveg.html) in 3513 adults found 2 % of respondents to be "completely vegetarian". The number of vegans in the UK is estimated to be at around 0.3 % of the population (180,000 people: www.imaner.net/panel/statistics.htm). Further reliable information based on the available research (Dietary Habits of Adults 18 and Older in the United States) puts the figure ranging from 0.5 % – 1.4 % of the USA population to be vegan, with the possible exception of honey (2006: www.vrg.org/journal/vj2006issue4/vj2006issue4poll.htm, 2008: www.imaner.net/panel/statistics.htm). The number of vegetarians – including vegans – in the USA is expected to increase during the next decade (2009b).

In general, vegetarians are known to be more *"health conscious"* than non-vegetarians (Bedford and Barr 2005). To date, the female MTB athlete has successfully followed a vegan lifestyle since 1999 and thus has gained previous experience.

According to the meta–analysis of the ADA (2003/2009a+b), a vegetarian – including vegan – diet can meet current recommendations for all nutrients. A well planned vegan and other type of vegetarian diet is appropriate for all stages of the life cycle, including during pregnancy, lactation, infancy, childhood and adolescence, and for athletes. Vegetarian diets offer a number of nutritional benefits as well as higher levels of CHOs.

"It is the position of the American Dietetic Association that appropriately planned vegetarian diets, including vegetarian or vegan diets, are healthful, nutritionally adequate, and may provide health benefits in the prevention and treatment of certain diseases" (ADA 2009b).

Together, these advantages include lower risk for heart disease, blood cholesterol levels, blood pressure, hypertension, diabetes mellitus, obesity and some types of cancer (ADA 2003/2009b, Campbell and Campbell 2006, Kugler 2007, Venderly and Campbell 2006).

After many years of research, mainly focused on issues connected to health (nutritional adequacy and the implications for diseases of affluence) rather than on human performance issues, the effects of a plant based diet on athletic performance are still unclear. Little is know about the relationship between vegetarianism and athletic performance even today, in spite of the popular belief that these kinds of diet may be beneficial to some athletes. Thus, there is a certain lack of information relating to veganism and its relationship to endurance performance. All athletes at some time in their career look at alternative eating patterns in the effort to reach their full athletic potential. While some take pills and/or powders, others have changed their nutritional styles to a vegetarian diet to gain advantages in training and enhance performance (Berning 2002).

However, any athlete, regardless of whether omnivore or vegan, should plan his/her diet carefully to avoid the risk of nutritional deficiencies and adverse effects on performance (Berning 2002, Venderly and Campbell 2006). There is sufficient evidence from laboratory and field that a well planned vegetarian or vegan diet can meet the energy and nutrient requirements of a competitive athlete (ADA 2003/2009a+b, Barr and Rideout 2004, Venderly and Campbell 2006). The current findings confirm that this challenge can be met when the subject follows a well planned and monitored vegan diet.

As mentioned before, CHO is the vital fuel during prolonged intensive endurance exercise (Burke 2001, Jeukendrup 2002a+b). It is broadly accepted that endurance athletes involved in heavy endurance training and competition should ingest a higher amount of energy from CHO to maximize muscle glycogen synthesis. Niemann (1988) suggested that particularly those athletes training for more than 60 – 90 min/day should consume 60 – 70 % of their energy from CHO.

The main advantages of vegetarian diets are the higher amounts of CHO, including numerous higher CHOs, lower fat and adequate protein (ADA 2003/2009a+b, Niemann 1988, Venderly and Campbell 2006). Vegans in particular consume the majority of their energy from CHO (Messina and Messina 1996, Venderly and Campbell 2006). Messina and Messina (1996) summarizing dietary data from 63 studies, reported that among the general public, the CHO intake of vegans ranges from 50 – 65 % of total daily energy. Therefore, endurance athletes might adopt vegetarian diets as an optimum strategy in order to meet increased CHO needs and to assist in weight control (Cox 2000, Niemann 1988).

The formerly common opinion that a vegetarian diet is not advisable for athletes due to a small amount of high quality protein, cannot be hold nowadays. Appropriate protein provision is met by adopting a well–planned vegan diet (Williams 1997). With respect to the quality of animal protein repeatedly attested to in the literature as being "high", this level of quality has to be fundamentally questioned from a nutritional point of view. Meat, fish, egg and dairy products are produced by the commercial sector of livestock and animal farming industries. In order to maximize profits, processes aimed at the reaching of economic goals are often targeted at the practices within animal farming industries. Because the physiological units would not survive the conditions in life stocking, the production process has to be supported by the use of medical substances and supplements such as antibiotics, growth hormones, psychotropics and tranquillizers, which is commonly practice in animal farming industries. As a consequence, the excessive dose of medical treatment cannot be catabolized within very short lifetimes. Thus, a cocktail of residues from medical substances is contained within any kind of animal protein, as documented by numerous independent laboratories, widely known.

Research indicates that vegan competitive athletes can meet protein requirements exclusively from plant based sources (which provide all essential amino acids and ensure adequate nitrogen retention) when a variety of plant foods is consumed and energy needs are met (ADA 2003/2009a+b). Due to the diminished digestibility of plant protein, the requirement of protein is classified to be 20 – 30 % higher than with an omnivore diet (Kugler 2007). However, typical protein intakes of vegans (10 – 12 % of EI) appear to meet and exceed requirements (ADA 2009b, Barr and Rideout 2004, Kugler 2007, Larson 2000, Messina and Messina 1996), without the use of special foods or supplements (Larson 2000). Figure 26 depicts an overview of macronutrient intake reported and recommended in literature.

During the TAC 2004, the mean daily intakes of CHO and protein were found to meet or exceed recommended levels through a well planned vegan diet.

Figure 26. Breakdown of macronutrients as a percentage of total energy intake according to type of activity or sports (derived from available literature). Norm = normal distribution of general population. Vegan = distribution of vegans (non–athletes). Endurance cycling = endurance cyclists (Tour de France, Vuelta a Espana, competitive endurance cyclists and athletes). RAAM = Race Across America. TAC 2004 = Transalp Challenge 2004. ₁(Venderly and Campbell 2006), ₂(Messina and Messina 1996), ₃(Gabel 2002, Garcia–Roves et. al. 1998, Geiss and Hamm 1992, Niemann 1988, Saris et. al. 1989), ₄(Knechtle et. al. 2005, Lindemann 1991), ₅(Wirnitzer, 2009a+b). CHO = carbohydrate.

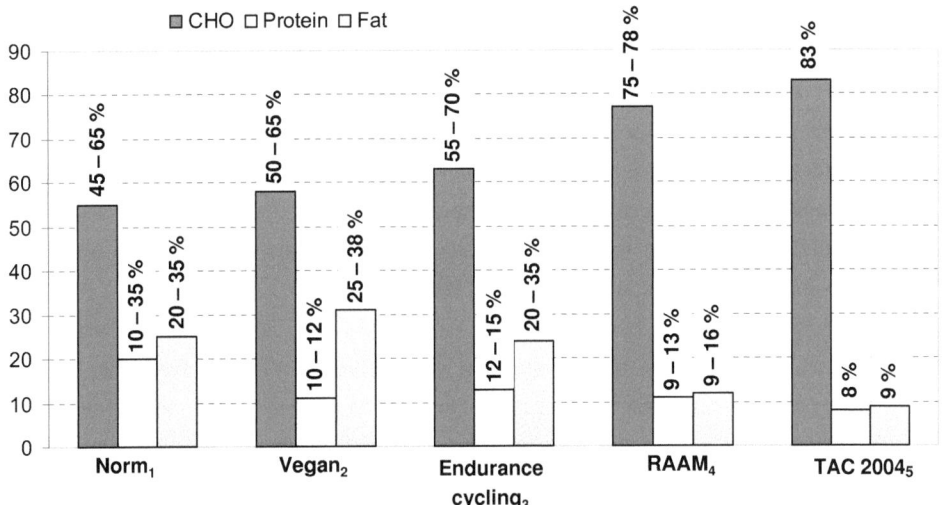

Iron status. Key nutrients for adolescent vegetarians include calcium, iron, zinc, vitamin D and B 12. A well planned vegan diet does not cause a deficiency in any of these nutrients when energy needs are met (ADA 2003, Kugler 2007).

Concerns about the iron status of vegetarian athletes are usually based on the bioavailability of iron from plant foods rather than the amount of total iron present in a vegetarian diet (Sabate et. al. 1999/2001). Shaw et. al. (1995) found in a comparative study that daily iron intake was similar in both vegetarian and non–vegetarian men, but iron intake was significantly higher in female vegetarians than non–vegetarians. It has been found that vegans can compensate for a diminished ingestion of calcium and iron by an adaptation of metabolism in both increased absorption and decreased losses (ADA

2009a+b, Hunt and Roughead 1999/2000, Kugler 2007). Saris et. al. (1989) found high EI resulting in high calcium and iron intake during the Tour de France.

Since iron plays a critical role in oxidative energy metabolism, it is vital for endurance athletes to have adequate iron stores. It is used for the synthesis of hemoglobin and myoglobin, essential components in the transport and delivery of oxygen to muscles (Sabate et. al. 1999). Generally, endurance training and competition tend to reduce iron stores (ADA 2003). Messina and Messina (1996) reported that only 10 % of athletes have anaemia and that it is more commonly found among endurance athletes. In general, iron deficiency anaemia is rare in vegetarian athletes, but is commonly reported in female athletes (Niemann 1999, Venderly and Campbell 2006). Therefore, it is especially important to monitor iron status especially in endurance and female athletes (ADA 2009a).

However, iron deficiency is observed in 20 % of the world population, with a similar incidence of iron deficiency amongst vegetarians or vegans as amongst omnivores (ADA 2003/2009b, Kugler 2007). Vegan and omnivore athletes alike must consume sufficient iron to prevent deficiency, which will adversely affect performance. In general, vegetarian diets contain as much or more total iron than omnivore diets and is usually highest in vegans (ADA 2003, Messina and Messina 1996).

A late and severe period of training close to the TAC 2004 resulted in a trend of lower iron levels. Despite this, the pre race levels of iron, ferritin and vitamin B 12 were within a normal range in the female subject (Table 9). In order to prevent an iron deficiency which might have resulted in a reduced aerobic capacity during the subsequent stage race, the female was treated by an intravenous application of iron supplement on 10 occasions including 100 mg of iron each (surgery). Sobal and Marquart (1994), reviewing 51 studies (10274 athletes), found a supplement use in female athletes of 57 %. Vitamin and mineral supplementation (orally or by intravenous injection) is common practice during professional tour races, especially after hard stages (Lucia et. al. 2003b, Saris et. al. 1989), which ensures a daily micronutrient intake considerably higher than the recommended daily allowance, especially for iron and vitamin B 12 (Saris et. al. 1989).

Despite the frequently proven benefits on health, sports scientists still doubt the advantageous effects of vegetarian diets on performance (ADA 2003), although an impressive number of high performance athletes (world record holders, national and international champions, attendants in World Championships, Olympic Games and World Cup, winners and multiple winners of major cycling tours etc.) from several disciplines such as marathon running, triathlon and ironman as well as cycling (including MTB sports) confirm the positive benefits for endurance performance.

Since professional cyclists like Adam Myerson (road–cycling), Christine Vardaros (cyclo–cross), Jason Sager (MTB), Sally Hibberd (British Women MTB Champion), Estelle Gray and Cheryl Marek (hold the world record for cross–country tandem cycling) and professional triathletes (ironman winners and finishers) like Brendan Brazier, Lucy Stephens and Ruth Heidrich have all adopted a vegan nutrition pattern (www.organicathlete.org/pro–activist, www.organicathlete.org/search/node/pro–activist, www.veganfitness.net/forum/viewtopic.php?t=723), the vegan diet has been demonstrated to be adequate for high performance events due to the advantageous effects on prolonged and high intensive endurance performance.

Limitations of this case report. The food diary is commonly used in most self–reported dietary surveys to monitor the intake during a specific event. Burke (2001) concluded in her review that dietary surveys during the racing practices of high level endurance cyclists provide a potential source of important information.

Unfortunately, inaccuracies due to several factors (memory failure, frequency of consumption, estimating portion size by not weighing the mass of food) are a universal problem (Burke 2001, Jeukendrup 2002b). This might result in considerable errors, leading to underestimate or overestimate intake ranging from 20 – 50 % (Burke 2001, Jeukendrup 2002b).

However, the most accurate self–reports might be expected to be derived from athletes who are confident of their eating habits, aware of their body image and who are highly motivated to receive valuable feedback (Burke 2001). As mentioned before, the subject is highly self–aware, a very experienced vegan. Thus, the nutritional strategy during the TAC 2004 was carefully planned and accurately accomplished in order to minimize and control for the errors involved in the survey techniques described in the method section. Therefore, EI is probably not biased by either self–report or race tactics (bunch building and/or drafting). Considering the former case reports on dietary pattern comparable to this case study (Knechtle et. al. 2005, Lucia et. al. 2003b) the error of EI might be similar to those or perhaps of a considerably lesser magnitude. However, the author is absolutely aware that the use of self–reported dietary survey to determine the EI of a specific event is potentially limited. Since no indicators of dietary intake free from potential limitations exist, the use of self–reported dietary surveys can be acceptable for quantifying the EI in the present case report under authentic race burden of the TAC 2004.

4.4. Mood and mental capacity

Factors other than aerobic and anaerobic power and capacity, off–road cycling economy, technical ability and nutritional strategies amongst others, might influence MTB performance (Impellizzeri and Marcora 2007, Impellizzeri et. al. 2008). Optimum physiological preparation alone does not lead to winning a race.

Differences in HR_{MAX} determined in laboratory versus field setting may be due to a number of reasons, including psychological motivation of the athlete to really push himself/herself to his/her maximum capacity, or the duration of an event. Results of Foster et. al. (1993) and Palmer (2002) suggest that under competitive conditions with athletes free to regulate PO on a moment by moment basis, greater physiological responses may be achieved than when work pattern is dictated by laboratory protocol.

Mood status and mental strength are of vital importance for success when participating in XCM, ultraendurance and stage races. When two cyclists are at the top of their performance level, how they can push themselves and deal with the psychological factors and mental situation can decide between victory or defeat, coming first or second (Häuser et. al. 1991, Handow 2003, Johnson et. al. 1985, Rauch et. al. 1988, Schlicht et. al. 1989a+b+c/1990a+b, Seiler 1995). Because of this fact it was decided to include a further Smilie (value 2 = good) within the questionnaire (see Figure 2) to support a better interpretation of results.

When strenuous prolonged exercise is conducted under hot and dry conditions, in particular under authentic race burdens as during the TAC 2004, the mental situation is heavily stressed. High tolerance of heat, fatigue of muscle groups recruited (mainly leg muscles) as well as impaired mood status and mental situation, are all necessary to successfully perform at a high level. Significant dehydration has been found to result in diminished mental performance, in particular in reduced problem solving ability and diminished visual–motor tracking (Gopinathan et. al. 1988, Sawka et. al. 2007, Sharma et. al. 1986), which is of premium importance for the downhill performance capacity during strenuous and exertive MTB races where single trails are usually technically very difficult and challenging.

5. Conclusion

To the best of the author's knowledge there have been no published studies investigating MTB marathon races, 1–day UCI XCM races or MTB stage races yet been published. Moreover, well controlled long term studies assessing the effects of a vegan diet to athletes performance, in particular endurance performance, have not yet been conducted.

This report was the first to

i) describe the exercise intensity during one of the most important MTB stage races in the world, showing the TAC 2004 to be physiologically very demanding and heavily involving both the aerobic and anaerobic energy system,
ii) study a female MTBer during this difficult multi–day XCM competition and
iii) report the dietary intake during the TAC 2004, showing that a well planned vegan diet can adequately meet the nutritional demands of severe MTB stage racing.

The current findings might be useful to design specific training programs and to develop appropriate nutritional strategies to sustain the physical demands of severe XCM and MTB stage races. Therefore, prospective research should aim to focus on 1–day MTB XCM and MTB stage events, female off–road cyclists as well as vegetarian and vegan dietary patterns and their influence on endurance performance, particularly on high performance (road and off–road) cycling and stage racing.

References

American Dietetic Association, Dietitians of Canada (ADA) (2003) Position of the American Dietetic Association and Dietitians of Canada. Vegetarian diets. *J Am Diet Assoc* 103(6): 748 – 765

American Dietetic Association, Dietitians of Canada, and the American College of Sports Medicine (ADA) (2009a) Position of the American Dietetic Association, Dietitians of Canada, and the American College of Sports Medicine. Nutrition and Athletic Performance. *J Am Diet Assoc* 109(4): 509 – 527

American Dietetic Association (ADA) (2009b) Position of the American Dietetic Association: Vegetarian diets. *J Am Diet Assoc* 109(7): 1266 – 1282

Astrand P–O (1968) Something old and something new ... very new. *Nutrition Today* 3(2): 9 – 11

Auferbauer R (2007) Am Anfang war der Berg. *RADWELT* 04/2007: 54 – 58. St. Pölten: GEPA

Baron R (2001) Aerobic and anaerobic power characteristics of off–road cyclists. *Med Sci Sports Exerc* 33(8): 1387 – 1393

Barr SI, Rideout CA (2004) Nutritional Considerations for vegetarian athletes. *Nutrition* 20(7–8): 696 – 703

Bedford JL, Barr SI (2005) Diets and selected lifestyle practices of self–defined adult vegetarians from a population–based sample suggest they are more 'health conscious'. *Int J Behav Nutr Phys Act* 2(1): 4

Below PR, Mora–Rodriguez R, Gonzalez–Alonso J, Coyle EF (1995) Fluid and carbohydrate ingestion independentely improve performance during 1 h of intense exercise. *Med Sci Sports Exerc* 27(2): 200 – 210

Beneke R (1998) Belastungsempfinden nach Borg auch von der Sportart abhängig? In: *Sportpsychologische Diagnostik, Prognostik, Intervention* – Reihe: Psychologie & Sport, Band 34: 149 – 153

Berning JR (2002) The Vegetarian Athlete. In: Maughan RJ (ed) *Nutrition in Sport. Part 2: Special Considerations.* Chapter 33: 442 – 456. Oxford: Blackwell Science

Berry E (1909) The effects of a high and low protein diet on physical efficiency. *Am Phys Ed Rev* 14: 288 – 297

Berry MJ, Koves TR, Benedetto JJ (2000) The influence of speed, grade and mass during simulated off road bicycling. *Appl Ergon* 31(5): 531 – 536

Borg G (1982) Ratings of perceived exertion and heart rates during short–term cycle exercise and their use in a new cycling strength test. *J Sports Med* 3(3): 153 – 158

Borg G (1998) The Borg RPE Scale. In: Borg G (ed) *Borg`s perceived exertion and pain scales*. Chapter 5: 29 – 38. Champaign: Human Kinetics

Borg G (2004) Anstrengungsempfinden und körperliche Aktivität. *Deutsches Ärzteblatt* 101(15): A1016 – A1021

Brouns FJ, Saris WH, ten Hoor F (1986) Dietary problems in the case of strenuous exertion. *J Sports Med Phys Fitness* 26(3): 306 – 319

Brouns F, Saris WHM, Stroecken J, Beckers JE, Thijssen R, Rherer NJ, ten Hoor F (1989a) Eating, drinking and cycling. A controlled Tour de France simulation study, Part I. *Int J Sports Med* 10(Suppl): S32 – S40

Brouns F, Saris WHM, Stroecken J, Beckers JE, Thijssen R, Rherer NJ, ten Hoor F (1989b) Eating, drinking and cycling. A controlled Tour de France simulation study, Part II. Effect of diet manipulation. *Int J Sports Med* 10(Suppl): S41 – S48

Buchholz AC, Bartok C, Schöller DA (2004) The validity of bioelectrical impedance models in clinical populations. *Nutr Clin Pract* 19(5): 433 – 446

Burke LM (2001) Nutritional practices of male and female endurance cyclists. *Sports Med* 31(7): 521 – 532

Burke LM (2002) Principles of Eating for Cycling. In: Jeukendrup AE (ed) *High–Performance Cycling. Part IV: Nutrition*. Chapter 16: 183 – 200. Champaign: Human Kinetics

Campbell TC, Campbell TM (2006) *The China Study. Startling implications for diet, weight loss and long–term health*. Part I: The China Study: 27 – 31, 43 – 67 and Part II: Diseases of Affluence: 109 – 225. Dallas, Texas: BenBella

Chittenden RH (1904) *Physiological economy in nutrition*. New York: F. A. Stokes

Chittenden RH (1907) *The nutrition of man*. New York: F. A. Stokes

Christensen EH, Hansen O (1939a) Arbeitsfähigkeit und Ernährung. *Scand Arch Physiol* 81: 160 – 171

Christensen EH, Hansen O (1939b) Hypoglykämie, Arbeitsfähigkeit und Ermüdung. *Scand Arch Physiol* 81: 172 – 179

Coggan AR, Coyle EF (1987) Reversal of fatigue during prolonged exercise by carbohydrate infusion or ingestion. *J Appl Physiol* 63(6): 2388 – 2395

Coggan AR, Coyle EF (1988) Effect of carbohydrate feeding during high–intensity exercise. *J Appl Physiol* 65(4): 1703 – 1709

Coggan AR, Coyle EF (1989) Metabolism and performance following carbohydrate ingestion late in exercise. *Med Sci Sports Exerc* 21(1): 59 – 65

Convertino VA, Greenleaf JE, Bernauer EM (1980) Role of thermal and exercise factors in the mechanism of hypervolemia. *J Appl Physiol* 48(4): 657 – 664

Convertino VA (1983) Heart rate and sweat rate responses associated with exercise–induced hypervolemia. *Med Sci Sports Exerc* 15(1): 77 – 82

Convertino VA (1991) Blood volume: Its adaption to endurance training. *Med Sci Sports Exerc* 23(12): 1338 – 1348

Cox G (2000) Special needs: the vegetarian athlete. In: Burke L, Deakin V (ed) *Clinical sports nutrition.* Chapter 20: 656 – 671. Sydney, NSW: McGraw–Hill

Coyle EF, Feltner ME, Kautz SA (1991) Physiological and biomechanical factors associated with elite endurance cycling performance. *Med Sci Sports Exerc* 23(1): 93 – 107

Cramp T, Broad E, Martin D, Meyer BJ (2004) Effects of preexercise carbohydrate ingestion on mountain bike performance. *Med Sci Sports Exerc* 36(9): 1602 – 1609

De Marees H (2003) *Sportphysiologie.* Kapitel 10.2.2.7: Elektrolyt– und Wasserbedarf des Sportlers: 421 – 424. Korrigierter Nachdruck der 9., vollständig überarbeiteten und erweiterten Auflage. Köln: Verlag Sport & Buch Strauß

Dietary Habits of Adults 18 and Older in the United States 2006. Available from URL: www.vrg.org/journal/vj2006issue4/vj2006issue4poll.htm (5. 8. 2009)

Eichner ER (1992) Sports anemia, iron supplements, and blood doping. *Med Sci Sports Exerc* 24(9Suppl): S315 – S318

Erp van–Baart AM, Saris WH, Binkhorst RA, Vos JA, Elvers JWH (1989) Nationwide survey on nutritional habits in elite athletes. Part I. Energy, carbohydrate, protein. *Int J Sports Med* 10(Suppl)1: S3 – S10

Faria EW, Parker DL, Faria IE (2005a) The science of cycling: physiology and training – part 1. *Sports Med* 35(4): 285 – 312

Faria EW, Parker DL, Faria IE (2005b) The science of cycling: Factors affecting performance – part 2. *Sports Med* 35(4): 313 – 337

Febbraio MA (2002) Exercise in climatic extremes. In: Maughan RJ (ed) *Nutrition in Sport. Part 3: Practical Issues.* Chapter 38:497 – 509. Oxford: Blackwell Science

Fellmann N (1992) Hormonal and plasma volume alterations following endurance exercise. A brief review. *Sports Med* 13(1): 37 – 49

Fellmann N, Ritz P, Rubeyre J, Beazfrere B, Delaitre M, Coudert J (1999) Intracellular hyperhydration induced by a 7–day endurance race. *Eur J Appl Physiol Occup Physiol* 80(4): 353 – 359

Fernandez–Garcia B, Perez–Landaluce J, Rodriguez–Alonso M, Terrados N (2000) Intensity of exercise during road race pro–cycling competition. *Med Sci Sports Exerc* 32(5): 1002 – 1006

Fisher I (1907) The Influence of Flesh Eating on Endurance. *Yale Medical Journal* 13(5): 205 – 211

Food Standards Agency. Consumer Attitudes to Food Standards 2007. Available from URL: www.vegsoc.org/info/statveg.html (5. 8. 2009)

Foster C, Snyder AC, Thompson NN, Green MA, Foley M, Schrager M (1993) Effect of pacing strategy on cycle time trial performance. *Med Sci Sports Exerc* 25(3): 383 – 388

Gabel KA (2002) The Female Athlete. In: Maughan RJ (ed) *Nutrition in Sport. Part 2: Special Considerations.* Chapter 31: 417 – 428. Oxford: Blackwell Science

Galloway SDR, Maughan RJ (2000) The effects of substrate and fluid provision on thermoregulatory and metabolic responses to prolonged excercise in a hot environment. *J Sports Sci* 18(5): 339 – 351

Galy O, Hue O, Boussana A, Peyreigne C, Mercier J, Prefaut C (2005) Blood rheological responses to running and cycling: A potential effect on the arterial hypoxemia of highly trained athletes? *Int J Sports Med* 26(1): 9 – 15

Garcia–Roves PM, Terrados N, Fernandez SF, Patterson AM (1998) Macronutrients intake of top level cyclists during continuous competition – change in the feeding pattern. *Int J Sports Med* 19(1): 61 – 67

Garcin M, Vautier JF, Vandewalle H, Monod H (1998a) Ratings of perceived exertion (RPE) as an index of aerobic endurance during local and general exercises. *Ergon* 41(8): 1105 – 1114

Garcin M, Vautier JF, Vandewalle H, Wolff M, Monod H (1998b) Ratings of perceived exertion (RPE) during cycling exercises at constant power output. *Ergon* 41(10): 1500 – 1509

Geiss K–R and Hamm M (1992) *Handbuch Sportlerernährung.* Überarbeitete Neuausgabe. Kapitel 2.2: Energieumsatz: 17 – 19 und Kapitel 4.2.5: Ausdauersportarten: 190 – 191. Reinbeck, Hamburg: Rowolth Taschenbuch Verlag, Sport rororo

Gerig U, Frischknecht T (1996) Mountainbiking. In: Weiss C (ed) *Handbuch Radsport.* Mountainbiking: 323 – 326. München: BLV Verlagsgesellschaft mbH

Gilman MB, Wells CL (1993) The use of heart rates to monitor exercise intensity in relation to metabolic variables. *Int J Sports Med* 14(6): 339 – 344

Gilman MB (1996) The use of heart rate to monitor the intensity of endurance training. *Sports Med* 21(2): 73 – 79

Gopinathan PM, Pichan G, Sharma VM (1988) Role of dehydration in heat–stress induced variations in mental performance. *Arch Environ Health* 43(1): 15 – 17

Gregory J, Johns DP, Walls JT (2007) Relative vs. Absolute physiological measures as predictors of mountain bike cross–country race performance. *J Strength Cond Res* 21(1): 17 – 22

Grund A, Krause H, Kraus M, Siewers M, Rieckert H, Muller MJ (2001) Association between different attributes of physical activity and fat mass in untrained, endurance– and restistance–trained men. *Eur J Appl Physiol* 84(4): 310 – 320

Guglielmini C, Casoni I, Patracchini M, Manfredini F, Grazzi G, Ferrari M, Conconi F (1989) Reduction of Hb levels during the racing season in nonsideropenic professional cyclists. *Int J Sports Med* 10(5): 352 – 356

Häuser W, Urhausen A, Welsch P (1991) Psychische Bewältigung eines (Ultra–) Langtriathlon. *Deutsche Zeitschrift für Sportmedizin* 42(8): 336 – 350

Hagberg JM, Coyle EF (1983) Physiological determinants of endurance performance as studied in competitive race walkers. *Med Sci Sports Exerc* 15(4): 287 – 289

Handow O (2003) Das Rennen wird im Kopf entschieden – Psychologische Maßnahmen in den verschiedenen Phasen eines Marathons. *Condition* 34(1–2): 40 – 41

Hardinge MG, Crooks H (1963) Non–flesh dietaries II. Scientific literature. *J Am Diet Assoc* 43: 550 – 558

Hargreaves M, Costill DL, Coggan A, Fink WJ, Nishibata I (1984) Effect of carbohydrate feedings on muscle glycogen utilization and exercise performance. *Med Sci Sports Exerc* 16(3): 219 – 222

Hargreaves M, Dillo P, Angus D, Howlett K, Febbraio M (1996a) Effect of fluid ingestion on muscle metabolism during prolonged exercise. *J Appl Physiol* 80(1): 363 – 366

Hargreaves M, Angus D, Howlett K, Conus NM, Febbraio M (1996b) Effect of heat stress on glucose kinetics during exercise. *J Appl Physiol* 81(4): 1594 – 1597

Hargreaves M (2002) Carbohydrate Replacement during Exercise. In: Maughan RJ (ed) *Nutrition in Sport. Part 1: Nutrition and Exercise.* Chapter 8: 112 – 118. Oxford: Blackwell Science

Harrison MH (1985) Effects of thermal stress and exercise on blood volume in humans. *Physiol Rev* 65(1): 149 – 209

Hunt JR, Roughead ZK (1999) Nonheme–iron absorption, fecal ferritin excretion, and blood indexes of iron status in women consuming controlled loacto–ovovegetarian diets for 8 wk. *Am J Clin Nutr* 69(5): 944 – 952

Hunt JR, Roughead ZK (2000) Adaptation of iron absorption in men consuming diets with high or low iron bioavailability. *Am J Clin Nutr* 71(1): 94 – 102

Hurst HT, Atkins S (2002) The physiological demands of downhill mountain biking as determined by heart rate monitoring. *Communication to the 7th Annual Congress of the European College of Sports Sciences*. Athens, Greece

Hurst HT, Atkins S (2006) Power output of field–based downhill mountain biking. *J Sports Sci* 24(10): 1047 – 1053

http://ec.europa.eu/food/animal/welfare/euro_barometer25_volA_en.pdf (5. 8. 2009)

http://ester.chemie.fu–berlin.de/cgi–bin/units?from=kcal&to=kJ&have=&want (15. 2. 2009)

Impellizzeri FM, Sassi A, Rodriguez–Alonso M, Mognoni P, Marcora SM (2002) Exercise intensity during off–road cycling competitions. *Med Sci Sports Exerc* 34(11): 1808 – 1813

Impellizzeri FM, Rampinini E, Sassi A, Mognoni P, Marcora SM (2005a) Physiological correlates to off–road cycling performance. *J Sports Sci* 23(1): 41 – 47

Impellizzeri FM, Marcora SM, Rampinini E, Mognoni P, Sassi A (2005b) Correlations between physiological variables and performance in high level cross country off road cyclists. *Br J Sports Med* 39(10): 747 – 751

Impellizzeri FM, Marcora SM (2007) The Physiology of Mountain Biking. *Sports Med* 37(1): 59 – 71

Impellizzeri FM, Ebert T, Sassi A, Menaspa P, Rampinini E, Martin DT (2008). Level ground and uphill cycling ability in elite female mountain bikers and road cyclists. *Eur J Appl Physiol* 102(3): 335 – 341

Ioteyko J, Kipiani V (1906) Societe Scientifique d`Hygiene Alimentaire et de l`Alimentation Rationelle de l`Homme. *Revue* 3: 114 – 207. Brussels

Ioteyko J, Kipiani V (1907) Leur résistance à la fatigue étudiée à l'ergographe, la durée de leurs réactions nerveuses, considérations énergétiques et sociales. *Enquête scientifique sur les végétariens de Bruxelles:* 50. Brussels: Henri Lamertin

Ioteyko J (1911) L'enfance végétarienne. *Enquête sur 170 enfants végétariens:* 85. Bruselles: Misch et Thron

Jameson C, Ring C (2000) Contributions of local and central sensations to the perception of exertion during cycling: Effects of work rate and cadence. *J Sports Sci* 18(4): 291– 298

Jentjens R (2002) Eating Strategies for Stage Races. In: Jeukendrup AE (ed). *High-Performance Cycling. Part IV: Nutrition.* Chapter 15: 173 – 182. Champaign: Human Kinetics

Jeukendrup AE, Van Diemen A (1998) Heart rate monitoring during training and competition in cyclists. *J Sports Sci* 16(Suppl): S91 – S99

Jeukendrup AE, Craig NP, Hawley JA (2000) The Bioenergetics of World Class Cycling. *J Sci Med Sport* 3(4): 414 – 433

Jeukendrup AE (2002a) Cycling. In: Maughan RJ (ed). *Nutrition in Sport. Part 4: Sport-specific Nutrition.* Chapter 43: 562 – 573. Oxford: Blackwell Science

Jeukendrup AE (ed) (2002b) *High performance Cycling. Part IV: Nutrition.* Chapter 12: 139 – 153. Champaign: Human Kinetics

Johnson A, Collins P, Higgins I, Harrington D, Connolly J, Dolphin C, McCreery M, Brady L, O'Brien M (1985) Psychological, nutritional and physical status of olympic road cyclists. *Br J Sports Med* 19(1): 11 – 14

Kleiner SM (1999) Water: an essential but overlooked nutrient. *J Am Diet Assoc* 99(2): 200 – 206

Knechtle B, Enggist A, Jehle T (2005) Energy turnover at the Race Across America (RAAM) – a case report. *Int J Sports Med* 26(6): 499 – 503

Koivula N, Hassem P (1998) Central, local and overall ratings of perceived exertion during cycling and running by women with an extermnal or internal locus of control. *J Gen Psychol* 125(1): 17 – 29

Koulmann N, Jimenez C, Regal D, Bolliet P, Launa JC, Savourey G, Melin B (2000) Use of bioelectrical impedance analysis to estimate body fluid compartments after acute variations of the body hydration level. *Med Sci Sports Exerc* 32(4): 857 – 864

Kugler HG (ed) (2007) *Vegetarisch essen – Fleisch vergessen. Ärztlicher Ratgeber für Vegetarier und Veganer.* Marktheidenfeld: Verlag DAS WORT GmbH

Kuipers H, Verstappen FT, Keizer HA, Geurten P, van Kranenburg G (1985) Variability of aerobic performance in the laboratory and its physiologic correlates. *Int J Sports Med* 6(4): 197 – 201

Kyle UG, Bosaeus I, De Lorenzo AD, Deurenberg P, Elia M, Gomez JM, Heitmann BL, Kent–Smith L, Melchior JC, Pirlich M, Scharfetter H, Schols AM, Pichard C (2004a) Composition of the ESPEN Working Group. Bioelectrical impedance analysis – part I: Review of priciples and methods. *Clin Nutr* 23(5): 1226 – 1243

Kyle UG, Bosaeus I, De Lorenzo AD, Deurenberg P, Elia M, Gomez JM, Heitmann BL, Kent–Smith L, Melchior JC, Pirlich M, Scharfetter H, Schols AM, Pichard C (2004b)

Composition of the ESPEN Working Group. Bioelectrical impedance analysis – part II: Utilization in clinical practice. *Clin Nutr* 23(6): 1430 – 1453

Larson DE (2000) Vegetarian athletes. In : Rosenblooom CA (ed) *Sports Nutrition. A Guide for the Professional Working with Active People*. 3rd edition. 405 – 425. Chicago, IL: American Dietetic Association, Sports, Cardiovascular, and Wellness Dietetic Practice Group

Lee H, Martin DT, Anson JM, Grundy D, Hahn AG (2002) Physiological characteristics of successful mountain bikers and professional road cyclists. *J Sports Sci* 20(12): 1001 – 1008

Lee H (2003) Competitive mountain bike and road cycling: physiological characteristics of athletes and demands of competition. *Masters thesis.* Chapter 3 and 4. University of Canberra, Australia

Leiper JB, Pitsiladis Y, Maughan RJ (2001) Comprasion of water turnover rates in men undertaking prolonged cycling exercise and sedentary men. *Int J Sports Med* 22(3): 181 – 185

Lemon PWR (1995) Do athletes need more dietary protein and amino acids? *Int J Sport Nutr* 5(Suppl): S39 – S61

Lesewitz H (2004) Große Welle. *BIKE. Das Mountainbike–Magazin* 4/2004: 16 – 24. München: Delius Klasing

Lesewitz H (2005) Massenbewegung. Hall of Fame. *BIKE. Das Mountainbike–Magazin* 6/2005: 176 – 177. München: Delius Klasing

Le Système International d'Unités. Available from both URL: www.bipm.org, www.bipm.org/en/CGPM/db/11/12/ (5. 8. 2009)

Lindemann AK (1991) Nutrient intake in an ultraendurance cyclist. *Int J Sport Nutr* 1(1): 79 – 85

Lucia A, Hoyos J, Carvajal A, Chicharro JL (1999) Heart rate response to professional road cycling: the Tour de France. *Int J Sports Med* 20(3): 167 – 172

Lucia A, Hoyos J, Perez M, Chicharro JL (2000) Heart rate and performance parameters in elite cyclists: a longitudinal study. *Med Sci Sports Exerc* 32(19): 1777 – 1782

Lucia A, Hoyos J, Santalla A, Earnest CP, Chicharro JL (2003a) Tour de France versus Vuelta a Espana: which is harder? *Med Sci Sports Exerc* 35(5): 872 – 878

Lucia A, Hoyos J, Santalla A, Earnest CP, Chicharro JL (2003b) Giro, Tour and Vuelta in the same season. *Br J Sports Med* 37(5): 457 – 459

MacRae H, Hise KJ, Allen PJ (2000) Effects of front suspension and dual suspension mountain bike systems on uphill performance. *Med Sci Sports Exerc* 32(7): 1276 – 1280

Martin MK, Martin DT, Collier GR, Burke LM (2002) Voluntary food intake by elite female cyclists during training and racing: influence of daily energy expenditure and body composition. *Int J Sport Nutr Exerc Metab* 12(3): 249 – 267

Martinoli R, Mohamed El, Maiolo C, Cianci R, Denoth F, Salvadori S, Iacopino L (2003) Total body water estimation using bioelectrical impedance: a metaanalysis of the data available in literature. *Acta Diabetol* 40(Suppl)1: S203 – S206

Mastroianni GR, Zupan MF, Chuba DM, Berger RC, Wile AL (2000) Voluntary pacing and energy cost of off–road cycling and running. *Appl Ergon* 31(5): 479 – 485

Maughan RJ, Whiting PH, Davidson RJ (1985) Estimation of plasma volume changes during marathon running. *Br J Sports Med* 19(3): 138 – 141

Maughan R (2002) Fluid Balance. In: Jeukendrup AE (ed). *High–Performance Cycling. Part IV: Nutrition.* Chapter 13: 155 – 166. Champaign: Human Kinetics

Maw GJ, Mackenzie IL, Comer DA, Taylor NA (1996) Whole–body hyperhydration in endurance–trained males determined using radionuclide dilution. *Med Sci Sports Exerc* 28(8): 1038 – 1044

Maw GJ, Mackenzie IL, Taylor NA (1998) Human body–fluid distribution during exercise in hot, temperate and cool environments. *J Acta Physiol Scand* 163(3): 297 – 304

Messina M, Messina V (1996) Vegetarian diets for athletes. In: Messina M, Messina V (ed). *The dietitian's guide to vegetarian diets: issues and applications.* Chapter 5: 124 – 135, Chapter 15: 354 – 367. Gaithersburg, MD: Aspen Publishers

Mischler I, Boirie Y, Gachon P, Pialoux V, Mounier R, Rousset P, Coudert J, Fellmann N (2003) Human albumin synthesis is increased by an ultra–endurance trial. *Med Sci Sports Exerc* 35(1): 75 – 81

Mounier R, Pialoux V, Mischler I, Coudert J, Fellmann N (2003) Effect of hypervolemia on heart rate during 4 days of prolonged exercise. *Int J Sports Med* 24(7): 523 – 529

Mujika I, Padilla S (2002) Event Selection. In: Jeukendrup AE (ed). *High–Performance Cycling. Part II: Performance Assessment.* Chapter 7: 79 – 90. Champaign: Human Kinetics

Nethery VM (2002) Competition between internal and external sources of information during exercise: Influence on RPE and the impact of exercise load. *J Sports Med Phys Fitness* 42(2): 172 – 178

Neumayr G, Pfister R, Mitterbauer G, Gänzer H, Joannidis M, Eibl G, Hörtnagl H (2002a) Short–term effects of prolonged strenuous endurance exercise on the level of haematocrit in amateur cyclists. *Int J Sports Med* 23(3): 158 – 161

Neumayr G, Pfister R, Mitterbauer G, Gänzer H, Sturm W, Eibl G, Hörtnagl H (2002b) Exercise intensity of cycle–touring events. *Int J Sports Med* 23(7): 505 – 509

Neumayr G, Pfister R, Mitterbauer G, Gänzer H, Sturm W, Hörtnagl H (2003a) Heart rate response to ultraendurance cycling. *Br J Sports Med* 37(1): 89 – 90

Neumayr G, Pfister R, Mitterbauer G, Gänzer H, Joannidis M, Eibl G, Hörtnagl H (2003b) Die physiologischen Auswirkungen eines Rad–Marathons auf das Plasmavolumen. *Deutsche Zeitschrift für Sportmedizin* 54(1): 12 – 16

Neumayr G, Pfister R, Mitterbauer G, Mauerer A, Hörtnagl H (2004) Effect of ultramarathon cycling on the heart rate in elite cyclits. *Br J Sports Med* 38(1): 55 – 59

Neumayr G, Pfister R, Hörtnagl H, Mitterbauer G, Prokop W, Joannidis M (2005) Renal function and plasma volume following ultramarathon cycling. *Int J Sports Med* 26(1): 2 – 8

Niemann DC (1988) Vegetarian dietary practices and endurance performance. *Am J Clin Nutr* 48(3Suppl): 754S – 761S

Niemann DC (1999) Physical fitness and vegetarian diets: Is there a relation? *Am J Clin Nutr* 70(3Suppl): 570S – 575S

Nishii T, Umemura Y, Kitagawa K (2004) Full suspension mountain bike improves off–road cycling performance. *J Sports Med Phys Fitness* 44(4): 356 – 360

Nose H, Mack GW, Shi X, Nadel ER (1988) Shift in body fluid compartments after dehydration in humans. *J Appl Physiol* 65(1): 318 – 324

O'Brien C, Young AJ, Sawka MN (2002) Bioelectrical impedance to estimate changes in hydration status. *Int J Sports Med* 23(5): 361 – 366

Padilla S, Mujika I, Orbananos J, Angulo F (2000) Exercise intensity during competition time trials in professional road cycling. *Med Sci Sports Exerc* 32(4): 850 – 856

Padilla S, Mujika I, Orbananos J, Santisteban J, Angulo F, Jose–Goiriena J (2001) Exercise intensity and load during mass–start stage races in professional road cycling. *Med Sci Sports Exerc* 33(5): 796 – 802

Padilla S, Mujika I, Santisteban J, Impellizzeri FM, Goiriena JJ (2008) Exercise intensity and load during uphill cycling in professional 3–week races. *Eur J Appl Physiol* 102(4): 431 – 438

Palmer GS, Hawley JA, Dennis SC, Noakes TD (1994) Heart rate responses during a 4–d cycle stage race. *Med Sci Sports Exerc* 26(10): 1278 – 1283

Palmer GS (2002) Field Testing. In: Jeukendrup AE (ed). *High–Performance Cycling. Part II: Performance Assessment.* Chapter 7: 91 – 99. Champaign: Human Kinetics

Peters EM (2003) Nutritional aspects in ultra–endurance exercise. *Curr Opin Clin Nutr Metab Care* 6(4): 427 – 434

Petter K, Pohlmann T (2007) Die große vegane Nährwerttabelle. Wien: Eigenverlag. Available from URL: www.veganity.com/GVNWT/Naehrwerttabelle.pdf (5. 8. 2009)

Phillips RL, Lemon FR, Beeson WL, Kzuma JW (1978) Coronary heart disease mortality among Seventh–Day Adventists with differing dietary habits: a preliminary report. *Am J Clin Nutr* 31(10Suppl): S191 – S198

Pialoux V, Mischler I, Mounier R, Gachon P, Ritz P, Coudert J, Fellmann N (2004) Effect of equilibrated hydration changes on total body water estimates by bioelectrical impedance analysis. *Br J Nutr* 91(1): 153 – 159

Pivarnik JM, Leeds EM, Wilkerson JE (1984) Effects of endurance exercise on metabolic water production and plasma volume. *J Appl Physiol* 56(3): 613 – 618

Prins L, Treblache E, Myburgh KH (2007) Field and laboratory correlates of performance in competitive cross–country mountain bikers. *J Sports Sci* 25(8): 927 – 935.

Rauch TM, Tharion WJ, Strowman SR, Shukitt BL (1988) Psychological factors associated with performance in the ultramarathon. *J Sports Med Phys Fitness* 28(3): 237 – 246

Richardson RS, Verstraete D, Johnson SC, Luetkemeier MJ and Stray–Gundersen J (1996) Evidence of a secondary hypervolemia in trained man following acute high intensity exercise. *Int J Sports Med* 17(4):243 – 247

Robertson RJ, Moyna NM, Sward KL, Millich NB, Godd FL, Thompson PD (2000) Gender comparison of RPE at absolute and relative physiological criteria. *Med Sci Sports Exerc* 32(12): 2120 – 2129

Robinson N, Schattenberg L, Zorzoli M, Mangin P, Saugy M (2005) Haematological analysis conducted at the departure of the Tour de France 2001. *Int J Sports Med* 26(3): 200 – 207

Rodriguez–Marroyo JA, Garcia–Lopez J, Avila C, Jimenez F, Cordova A, Villa–Vicente JG (2003) Intensity of exercise according to topography in professional cyclists. *Med Sci Sports Exerc* 35(7): 1209 – 1215

Rose SC, Peters EM (2008) Ad libitum Adjustments to Fluid Intake in cool Environmental Conditions Maintain Hydration Status in a Three–Day Mountain bike Race. *Br J Sports Med* 2008 Jun 6. (Epub ahead of print)

Sabate J, Duk A, Lee CL (1999) Publications trends of vegetarian nutrition articles in biomedical lieterature, 1966–1995. *Am J Clin Nutr* 70(3Suppl): 601S – 607S

Sabate J, Ratzin–Turner RA, Brown JE (2001) Vegetarian diets: descriptions and trends. In: Sabate J (ed) *Vegetarian Nutrition.* Section I, Chapter 1: Background – Vegetarian Diets: Descriptions and Trends: 3 – 17. Boca Raton, FL: CRC Press

Saris WHM, van Erp–Baart MA, Brouns F, Westerterp KR, ten Hoor F (1989) Study on food intake and energy expenditure during extreme sustained exercise: the Tour de France. *Int J Sports Med* 10(Suppl)1: S26 – S31

Saris EH, Senden JM, Brouns F (1998) What is a normal red–blood cell mass for professional cyclists? *Lancet (Letter)* 352(9142): 1758

Savard GK, Nielsen B, Laszczynska J, Larsen BE, Saltin B (1988) Muscle blood flow is not reduced in humans during moderate exercise and heat stress. *J Appl Physiol* 64(2): 649 – 657

Sawka MN, Convertino VA, Eichner ER, Schnieder SM, Young AJ (2000) Blood volume: Importance and adaptions to exercise training, environmental stresses and trauma/sickness. *Med Sci Sports Exerc* 32(2): 332 – 348

Sawka MN, Burke LM, Eichner ER, Maughan RJ, Montain SJ, Stachenfeld NS (2007) American College of Sports Medicine position stand. Exercise and fluid replacement. *Med Sci Sports Exerc* 39(2): 377 – 390

Scheele B, Grieshaber G (2007) Der kleine Unterschied. *BIKE. Das Mountainbike–Magazin* 10/2007: 59 – 61. München: Delius Klasing

Scheele B (2008) Die erste Transalp. *BIKE. Das Mountainbike–Magazin* 11/2008: 128. München: Delius Klasing

Schlicht W (1989a) Belastung, Beanspruchung und Bewältigung. 1. Teil: Theoretische Grundlagen. *Sportpsychologie* 2(2): 10 – 17

Schlicht W (1989b) Belastung, Beanspruchung und Bewältigung. 2. Teil: Ausgewählte Merkmale zur Beurteilung einer Beanspruchungs– oder Streßreaktion. *Sportpsychologie* 2(3): 11 – 18

Schlicht W (1989c) Belastung, Beanspruchung und Bewältigung. 3. Teil: Bewältigungskompetenz und Pyrrhussiege. *Sportpsychologie* 2(4): 13 – 17

Schlicht W, Meyer N, Janssen JP (1990a) Psychische Bewältigung belastender Ereignisse im Triathlon – eine Pilotstudie, 1. Teil. *Sportpsychologie* 3(1): 5 – 14

Schlicht W, Meyer N, Janssen JP (1990b) Psychische Bewältigung belastender Ereignisse im Triathlon – eine Pilotstudie, 2. Teil: Emotionale Beanspruchungsreaktion und angemessene Bewältigung. *Sportpsychologie* 3(2): 5 – 9

Schmidt W, Maassen N, Trost F, Boning D (1988) Training induced effects on blood volume, erythrocyte turnover and haemoglobin oxygen binding properties. *Eur J Appl Physiol Occup Physiol* 57(4): 490 – 498

Schmidt W, Maassen N, Tegtbur U, Braumann KM (1989) Changes in plasma volume and red cell formation after a marathon competition. *Eur J Appl Physiol Occup Physiol* 58(5): 453 – 458

Schmidt W, Biermann B, Winchenbach P, Lison S, Boning D (2000) How valid is the determination of hematocrit values to detect blood manipulations? *Int J Sports Med* 21(2): 133 – 138

Schumacher YO, Grathwohl D, Barturen JM, Wollenweber M, Heinricht L, Schmid A, Huber G, Keul J (2000) Haemoglobin, haematocrit and red blood cell indices in elite cyclists. Are the control values for blood testing valid? *Int J Sports Med* 21(5): 380 – 385

Schumacher YO, Schmid A, Grathwohl D, Bultermann D, Berg A (2002) Haematological indices and iron status in athlethes of various sports and performances. *Med Sci Sports Exerc* 34(5): 869 – 875

Schouteden H (1904) Ergographie de la main droite et de la main gauche. *Annales de la Societe Royale des Sciences Medicales et Naturelles de Bruxelles* Tome XIII: 1 – 28. Brussels, Belgium: Henri Lamertain

Segal KR (1996) Use of bioelectrical impedance analysis measurement as an evaluation for participation in sports. *Am J Clin Nutr* 6(Suppl): S469 – S471

Seifert JG, Luetkemeier MJ, Spencer MK, Miller D and Burke ER (1997) The effects of mountain bike suspension systems on energy expenditure, physical exertion and time trial performance during mountain bicycling. *Int J Sports Med* 18(3): 197 – 200

Seiler R (1995) Der Erfolg beginnt im Kopf! *Schweizerische Zeitschrift für Sportmedizin und Sporttraumatologie* 43(2): 25 – 31

Shanholtzer BA, Patterson SM (2003) Use of bioelectrical impedance in hydration status assessment: reliability of a new tool in psychophysiology research. *Int J Psychophysiol* 49(3): 217 – 226

Sharma VM, Sridharan K, Pichan G, Panwar MR (1986) Influence of heat–stress induced dehydration on mental functions. *Ergon* 29(6): 791 – 799

Shaw NS, Chin CJ, Pan WH (1995) A vegetarian diet rich in soybean products compromises iron status in young students. *J of Nutr* 125(2): 212 – 219

Sobal J, Marquart LF (1994) Vitamin/mineral supplement use among athletes: a review of the literature. *Int J Sport Nutr* 4(4): 320 – 334

Stapelfeldt B, Schwirtz A, Schumacher YO, Hillebrecht M (2004) Workload Demands in Mountain Bike Racing. *Int J Sports Med* 25(4): 294 – 300

Strauss MB, Davis RK, Rosenbaum JD, Rossmeisl EC (1951) Water diuresis produced during recumbency by the intravenous infusion of isotonic saline solution. *J Clin Invest* 30(8): 862 – 868

Takaishi T, Yasuda Y, Ono T, Moritani T (1996) Optimal pedalling rate estimated from neuromuscular fatigue for cyclists. *Med Sci Sports Exerc* 28(12): 1492 – 1497

Thomas BJ, Ward LC, Cornish BH (1998) Bioimpedance spectrometry in the determination of body water compartments: accuracy and clinical significance. *Appl Radiat Isot* 49(5–6): 447 – 455

Union Cycliste Internationale (UCI) (2009). Available from URL: www.uci.ch (5. 8 2009)

UCI Rules, Mountain Bike Races: Chapter I, II, VI, VIII, Annex, pages 1, 3, 6, 22, 24, 46: www.uci.ch/Modules/BUILTIN/getObject.asp?MenuId=MTkzNg&ObjTypeCode=FILE&type=FILE&id=34424& (5. 8 2009)

UCI XCM WC series: Available from URL: www.uci.ch/templates/UCI/UCI5/layout.asp?MenuId=MTUzNDI (5. 8 2009)

Venderly AM, Campbell WW (2006) Vegetarian Diets. Nutritional considerations for Athletes. *Sports Med* 36(4): 293 – 305

Vogt S, Heinrich L, Schumacher YO, Blum A, Roecker K, Dickhuth HH, Schmid A (2006) Power output during stage racing in professional road cycling. *Med Sci Sports Exerc* 38(1): 147 – 151

Von Liebig J (1842) *Animal chemistry*. Cambridge

Wang MJ, Hull ML (1997) A dynamic system model of an off–road cyclist. *J Biomech Eng* 119(3): 248 – 253

Warner SE, Shaw JM, Dalsky GP (2002) Bone mineral density of competitive male mountain and road cyclists. *Bone* 30(1): 281 – 286

Whorton JC (1982) *Crusaders for fitness*. Chapter Seven: Muscular Vegetarianism: 201 – 238. Princeton, NJ: Princeton University Press

Wilber RL, Zawadzki KM, Kearney JT, Shannon MP, Disalvo D (1997) Physiological profiles of elite off–road and road cyclists. *Med Sci Sports Exerc* 29(8): 1090 – 1094

Williams MH (1997) *Ernährung, Fintness und Sport*. Berlin/Wiesbaden: Ullstein Mosby

Wingo JE, Casa DJ, Berger EM, Dellis WO, Knight JC and McClung JM (2004) Influence of a Pre–Exercise Glycerol Hydration Beverage on Performance and Physiologic Function During Mountain–Bike Races in the Heat. *J Athl Train* 9(2): 169 – 175

Wirnitzer KC, Faulhaber M (2007) Hemoglobin and hematocrit during an 8 day mountainbike race: a field study. Letter to the Editor. *J Sports Sci Med* 6 (serial online). Available from both URL (5. 8. 2009): www.jssm.org/vol6/n2/16/v6n2-16text.php, www.jssm.org/vol6/n2/16/v6n2-16pdf.pdf

Wirnitzer KC, Kornexl E (2008) Exercise intensity during an eight–day mountain bike marathon race. *Eur J Appl Physiol* 104(6): 999 – 1005. © Full text article including figures (1, 2) and tables (1,2, 3) by courtesy of Springer Science and Business Media (14. 8. 2009).

Wirnitzer KC (2009a) Nutrition strategy during an eight–day mountainbike stage race – a case study. Vegan nutrition pattern of a female mountainbiker. Invited Book Chapter. In: *Aerobic Exercise: Types, Duration and Health Benefits.* Acceptance for publication confirmed on 18th February 2009 (release is scheduled to be published in 2009 4th quarter). New York, USA: Novapublishers. © Full text article including figures (1 – 13) and tables (1 – 6) by courtesy of Frank Columbus, Editor-in-Chief, Novapublishers (11. 9. 2009).

Wirnitzer KC (2009b) Athletic performance capacity in mountainbike sports with extremely strenuous more days lasting endurance impact. Performance determining and performance limiting factors during the Transalp Challenge. *Thesis.* University of Innsbruck, Austria. In extracts permanently available from URL: http://www.wirnitzer.at/da/thesis.pdf

www.bleibfit.at/kalorientabelle-naehrwerte.phtml, www.bleibfit.at (5. 8. 2009)

www.dge.de/modules.php?name=St&file=w_referenzwerte, www.dge.de (5. 8. 2009)

www.imaner.net/panel/statistics.htm (5. 8. 2009)

www.naehrwerttabelle.de (5. 8. 2009)

www.organicathlete.org/pro–activist (15. 2. 2009)

www.organicathlete.org/search/node/pro–activist (5. 8. 2009)

www.veganfitness.net/forum/viewtopic.php?t=723 (5. 8. 2009)

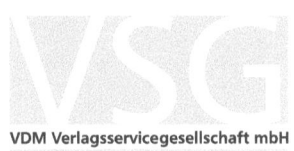

VDM Verlagsservicegesellschaft mbH

Die VDM Verlagsservicegesellschaft sucht für wissenschaftliche Verlage abgeschlossene und herausragende

Dissertationen, Habilitationen, Diplomarbeiten, Master Theses, Magisterarbeiten usw.

für die kostenlose Publikation als Fachbuch.

Sie verfügen über eine Arbeit, die hohen inhaltlichen und formalen Ansprüchen genügt, und haben Interesse an einer honorarvergüteten Publikation?

Dann senden Sie bitte erste Informationen über sich und Ihre Arbeit per Email an *info@vdm-vsg.de*.

Sie erhalten kurzfristig unser Feedback!

VDM Verlagsservicegesellschaft mbH
Dudweiler Landstr. 99   Telefon +49 681 3720 174
D - 66123 Saarbrücken   Fax   +49 681 3720 1749
www.vdm-vsg.de

Die VDM Verlagsservicegesellschaft mbH vertritt

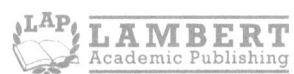
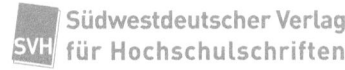

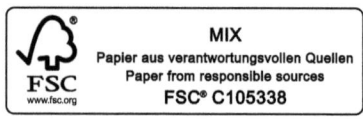

Printed by Books on Demand GmbH, Norderstedt / Germany